# VIRGIN SEX
## *for Girls*

## A NO-REGRETS GUIDE
## TO SAFE AND HEALTHY SEX

# Dr. Darcy Luadzers

**Hatherleigh Press**
**New York • London**

Hatherleigh Press
5-22 46th Avenue, Suite 200
Long Island City, NY 11101
www.hatherleighpress.com

CIP data available upon request.

ISBN-13: 978-1-57826-229-8
ISBN-10: 1-57826-229-1

Virgin Sex for Girls is available for bulk purchase, special promotions, and premiums. For information on reselling and special purchase opportunities, call 1-800-528-2550 and ask for the Special Sales Manager.

Interior design by Nancy Singer, and Deborah Miller
Cover design by Deborah Miller

10 9 8 7 6 5 4 3 2 1
Printed in Canada

# Contents

# Acknowledgments

Thank you to the many girls and women who courageously shared their true stories to help young women.

Thanks to my husband, Jack, for his endless support and patience throughout this project. From the late, late nights I stayed up to write and edit, while you took care of our children in the morning, to the discussion of many of the ideas presented in this book, over many nights. Thank you Jack, for your love and support over the years during the creation of this book.

Thank you to my children, Katie and Zack Marroso, and Dustin and Patrick Luadzers, who helped contribute to this book, through their experiences and expertise as teenagers, as well as their patience in listening to me when I said, "Don't bother me unless you're bleeding from the eyes."

A special thank you to my parents, Bob and Mary Fietsam, who read every word of my book, asked all the right questions, and did a very thorough job of last minute editing. Thank you, Dad, for the "Well Done," comment at the end of the book, with your signature. When choosing the title of the book, I struggled for weeks and many long hours over whether to call it "Virgin Sex," as I feared it was too bold and no parents would buy it for their teenager. My 65-year-old mother responded, "Well that's what it's about isn't it? It's not like you're using the "F" word on the cover!"

Thank you to my eight brothers and sisters: Dr. Bob Fietsam, Terry Fietsam, Wendy Gould, Cindy Matz, Randy Fietsam, Chad Fietsam, Skotti Gray, and Karolyn Tomayko. Thanks to my friends: Kitty

Mathis whose gourmet cooking kept me going, Caroline Tisdale, for her killer sense of humor, Deborah Genova and her daughters, Renee and Rachel, and all of my favorite friends from Folly Beach for their encouragement, helpful suggestions, and support.

Thank you to Jennifer Dechiara, my literary agent. I met Jennifer at the Book Expo in New York City, where I gave her a 30-second pitch on *Virgin Sex*, on the way to an elevator. She kindly gave me her time, listened, and said, "This is why I became an agent: to get this kind of book into the hands of teens." I thought I had died and gone to heaven. Jennifer understood my passion and purpose, why I wrote *Virgin Sex*: to help teens. Thank you, Jennifer, for your insight and vision, and creating one of the best days of my life when you agreed to represent me.

Books happen because publishers believe in authors and invest in a dream. Thank you to Hatherleigh Press, including my editors Andrea Au and Alyssa Smith, and Kevin Moran, the marketing director. A big thanks to Deborah Miller, the art director, with whom I had an amazingly fun and productive weekend shooting the Virgin Sex video.

A very special thank you to those very special people who took their precious, busy time to read the manuscript and make excellent suggestions: Bob Selverstone, an AASECT Certified Sex Educator, and Susan Humphrey, a sex educator at the Latin School in Chicago! Thank you to Sally A. Kope, my supervisor, and my mentor at AASECT. Thank you to Sallie Foley, my teacher and mentor from the University of Michigan: your sexuality class was the only course in my 22 years of education that I never missed, not even one day!

Last, but certainly not least, thank you, God, first of all, for inventing sex, but second for the strength, courage, and divine guidance to write and publish this book. With God's help, I hope that this book will find its way into the right girls' hands and heart at the right moments.

*To the many voices who joined as one*
*to send a powerful message among*
*young women everywhere, making a choice*
*while searching for their sexual voice*

*For my daughter, Katie, my girl, my heart.*

# A GIRL'S GUIDE FOR TEENS AND THEIR PARENTS!

Why is a girl's guide to sex so important? Because the combination of teens and sex is scary! Every day, as a sex therapist, I hear first hand accounts from people about sexual truths, sexual tragedies and sexual histories that start when girls were 12, 14, or 16, before they learned about safe and healthy sex. Often, a parent will call and ask about their child after a crisis, such as catching their 14-year-old daughter in her bed naked with her 17-year-old (did I mention he was naked, too?) boyfriend. The parent gets scared, calls hyperventilating, and asks "What do I do?" The answer is to give your daughter a guide to healthy sexuality, or talk with them about sex, or both. "How? What do I say? I just want to ground her for life and send the boy to jail!" Any parent can talk to their teen about sex, using my guide in Chapter 4, to talk to teens about what to know before they're really ready for sex. Parents and teens need straightforward guidance on helping teens make healthy and safe decisions about sex, which fit in with their family values about sexuality.

Why is a girl's guide to sex so important? Let's start with the facts and stats on teens and sex.

# The Truth About Teens and Sex

### On Sex

- 80% of teen girls engage in sexual activity
- One in 5 girls has sexual intercourse by age 15
- Nearly 50% of girls have sexual intercourse by the end of high school
- 50% of teens engage in oral sex, often as young as middle school
- 25% of girls say their first sexual experience was unwanted
- 90% of girls under 16 regret their first sexual experience

### On Pregnancy

- 1 in 12 teens get pregnant *every* year
- 1 in 5 sexually active teens gets pregnant
- 90% of girls who don't use birth control get pregnant within a year
- 33% of teen pregnancies end in abortion
- 80% of teen mothers are not married

### On Sexually Transmitted Diseases

- 1 out of 4 teen girls gets an STD
- 25% of new AIDS cases are young people under 21 years old
- 50% of new AIDS cases are young people under 25

(alanguttmacher.org, 2006, Division of Vital Statistics, 2005)

So, why do girls need a guide for sex? Girls need guidance to make the right choices, right from the start, and keep making choices about sex from the first time to the next time and every time. Girls need to have a sexual voice! A sexual voice is the most important ingredient to safe and healthy sex. Sex is not a single choice about the first time or about losing your virginity, it involves choices girls make in a part of their life that will be with them all of their life. Having a sexual voice and using it the first time and every time will help girls have fewer regrets about sex. Even if teens have already made some sexual choices, having a strong voice will help make better choices about saying yes or no or stop or go slow, from the beginning of one's sexual life and all throughout their sexual life. Even if a one make mistakes, which a lot of girls in this book have made, girls can always learn and become stronger, develop stronger sexual voices and have a safer, healthier love and life by makcr better decisions in the future.

*Virgin Sex* is about empowering girls to speak up for themselves and their sexual lives!

Although 80% of teens have sex, many stories are filled with regrets that girls have about their experiences with guys, when the girls wish they knew better, how to handle a situation better, or wish they "could turn back the hands of time." Many girls shared their very personal stories in *Virgin Sex*, with a hope that their story might help other girls avoid their mistakes, change the course of their lives, or change the hands of the future the next time, for someone else. This book is written for girls, some who are still virgins and some who are young and inexperienced but sexually active women. These true stories are the real lives that teens lead. They are secret stories other people don't hear about, don't know about, and maybe they'll never find out about, that lead them from adolescence to adulthood.

Sexual secrets shape lives forever. Sexual experiences, situations, and consequences shape the lives and futures of our daughters—and our friends, our sisters, or nieces, and granddaughters! As a sex therapist, I know what is really going on with teens and sex today, and I'm sure you would want your daughters to know what they need to know to be safe, sexually speaking. Every day in middle and high school, girls are getting sexually harassed. Every day after school our daughters are visiting friends, going to parties, hanging out, hooking up and some are getting sexually assaulted and raped. Every day girls are confused, worried and wondering how to deal with guys and what to do about "the sex thing." The sexual situations girls experience because they don't know better often affect them for life. Some young girls damage one of the precious gifts humans receive, their sexuality.

I wrote this book for teens because, at least once a day, someone comes into my office with an amazing complaint: they hate sex. Usually these are girls or women, many of them married, who don't know why they don't want to have sex even when they are totally in love with their partner and believe that they should be ready for sex in the relationship. Sex is supposed to be a playful, fun, and a magical connection between two people. Sadly, however, some people have sex problems as adults because they don't like sex, and some don't even like touching or other physical displays of affection. Some people feel like failures because it seems like everyone else is having and loving sex except them, and they believe there must be something deeply wrong with them. However, at some point early in their lives, most when they were teenagers, they learned to hate sex. This is nothing but a terrible disservice to these otherwise healthy women, because joyful sexual expression, when you are truly ready, is possible and a wondrous means for sharing one of most important things on Earth: love.

As a teenager, perhaps it is hard to imagine that there are people who hate sex, because sex is supposed to be a special celebration of love. Everyone simply knows this is true. Yet, every day I am saddened by the stories of first sexual experiences that were sad, scary, or traumatizing, and for a lot of different reasons. These experiences leave some women scarred by sex for their entire lives, regretting their first sexual experiences. When girls have sex for the wrong reasons, with the wrong person, in the wrong situation, in the wrong way, they can learn to hate sex. Girls who get hurt as teenagers by sex often lose their ability to love sharing one of the most special ways you can love another person: sharing love making and sharing your sexuality. With knowledge girls can search for the truth about who they are as a sexual person, for the first time and every time, in their life. Remember: knowledge is power and the foundation of wisdom.

Our society needs to change the way they treat teenagers when it comes to sex. As teens, our culture and media give girls two messages about sex: be beautiful, be hot, be sexy, get the guy, but say no to sex and don't get pregnant or you're a whore, a slut, ashamed, damaged goods. Teenagers are supposed to be sexually abstinent until they are married, and yet they are sexual people from birth. Teens have sexual feelings, they experience sexual situations, they have boyfriends, they fall in love, but, they aren't supposed to be sexual people until they are married, so real sex education remains a taboo subject. The reality is that the vast majority of teens have sexual experiences, but many girls have little or no sexual information on how to avoid getting hurt by sex. Girls need to know how to say no, how to know if a guy is going to hurt them or love them, how to handle themselves in relationships, how to make the right sexual choices, and how to be safe and healthy when they do act on their sexual feelings.

Girls need a guide *before* they try out their sexual ideas. Just like teens need driver's training *before* they get behind the wheel of a car, teens need sexual information *before* they start having closer, sexual relationships. Driver's education gives you a good foundation of knowledge about driving, signs, cars, directions, how to work the controls, and defensive driving so that reckless drivers don't hurt them. Teens use a few short weeks of education in driver's ed as a foundation of knowledge for their whole life. Girls need at least a few short weeks of education as a guide for sex, too.

When is the right time? Every state has different laws on what age is the right age to be able to legally drive. The average age is 15 or 16. Some teens are ready to take the wheel of a car at 15. But, many aren't. Even though they are legally able to drive, some parents won't let them get a beginner's permit or let them get a license, until they can show they are more responsible, like getting good grades, or following the rules in the home. Parents can be there and make that choice for kids about when they think their child is old enough to take on a responsibility to drive. Parents can have their kids pass tests, both written and driving tests, to prove that they are ready to drive and take their life into  their own hands, and be responsible for others' lives.

How does a parent know when is the time to put a kid into driving lessons? Some parents take their kids out driving at 12 or 13, long before it is "legal" to try to drive, usually on a farm or some back country roads or even the high school parking lot which is empty late at night or in the summer. How does a parent know when? Usually because a kid is asking to try it! "Let me hold the wheel" "Let me back the car out of the driveway" "When are you going to teach me to drive?" Teens won't ask parents "When are you going to tell me about sex?" "Let me tell you about making out in the driveway" "When can I start having sex?" Yet, long before it is "legal" for teens to have sex, at the age of consent, which might be age 16 (on average) or later, teens do take the "car out for a drive," and experiment sexually. Twenty-five percent of middle school kids have sexual experiences, through sexual touching and oral sex.

Parents can't always be there for teens when it comes to relationships and sex. Yet, knowledge and guidance set in place, set in motion, set in one's mind can never be taken away and can always be heard in the voices in one's mind, if they are placed in the right place in the right way, so they'll be heard. Parents don't give kids lessons on driving *after* they've wrecked the car: they give them lessons before an accident happens. Although knowledge won't prevent all accidents, it can prevent some, to learn to steer clear of dangerous situations and how to act in them when they happen, then learn to prevent them again in the future. When the time or situations arises where the sex drive is in gear, teens can be equipped to handle the road of relationships, some which will have sexual pitstops.

By using the "Dr. Darcy's Are You Ready for Sex" Quiz in Chapter 4, any parent can talk to their teens about sex, encouraging them to avoid sex until they can "pass" all the conditions needed to be ready for a sexual relationship. Parents might not be able to make their teens pass a test to be ready for sex, but they can give them the test as a guide to make the right decisions for sex. This guide isn't just a one time test one takes for a license to have sex the rest of their lives, it is a guide to use now and for the rest of their lives, when they are thinking about whether or not they are ready for sex in a particular situation, with a particular person, and at a particular time in their life.

When is the right time to give your teens a guide to sex? Before they have sexual touch, before they share oral sex, before they get pregnant, before they date and risk being date-raped, and before they get emotionally hurt by making sexual mistakes or before the next time or the next sexual decision. Twenty-five percent of girls are sexually assaulted or raped. Chapter 10 outlines specific ways to avoid sexual assault, before it happens, which is very important for every girl, especially college-bound girls, who are particularly vulnerable to date rape.

## Signs That Girls Need a Guide To Sex

- **Girls start talking to boys.**
- **Girls have interest in guys.**
- **Girls start chatting online with guys, privately.**
- **Guys start dropping by your house.**

- Girlfriends start chatting and talking about boys with each other.
- Girls start meeting with guys when they go out, like at the mall, the park, the school, the hang out place, the bowling alley, the local fast food place.
- Girls start talking to guys on the phone.
- The text messaging bill increases
- Guys start calling the house.
- "Trust" becomes a topic of conversation.
- Guys start hanging out at your house for hours at a time.
- When your child starts having secrets or lying about their whereabouts.

Virgin Sex is a guide for girls from 13 to 20. Some girls at 13 are still interested in primarily girl/girl activities, like playing games, riding bikes, and playing sports. But, when the interests turn to boys, it is time for girls to start understanding what sexuality is all about, to learn to speak up for themselves, and to develop a sexual voice. Girls need to learn to talk to guys and how to handle sexual situations. Sex starts with talking, then touching, then kissing and hugging, then sexual touch, then sexual talk, then sex. When girls start talking to guys and having interests in boy/girl relationships, it is time to start having serious talks or giving real sex education about sexuality. Many parents do not want to give their kids too much information because they think it will "give their child permission" to have sex. Research has found out that sex education does not make kids have sex earlier, in fact, it delays sexuality until later. Teens who participate in comprehensive sex education are more likely to act sexually responsibly by choosing abstinence or using protection against pregnancy and STDs. Sex education is effective in reducing unwanted pregnancies and STDs, not to mention the emotional pain from sexual mistakes. *Virgin Sex* encourages delaying sex until girls are ready for sex and to consider all the consequences and responsibilities of sexual behavior.

*Virgin Sex* will tell REAL, TRUE stories of teen sexual experiences and some of the many struggles that are seen in a sex therapist's office that happen in real life. The names of most of the girls and women have been changed, or the tellers of these stories have chosen names for themselves, to protect their identity. Some of the identifying circumstances have also been slightly altered to protect the identity of people in the stories, but some of the storytellers decided to use their real names and real details of their experiences to help get the truth out. Thanks is given to all the women who have had the courage to tell their true stories to help girls, the young reader of this book, to overcome fears and misgivings, to empower girls with knowledge, avoid negative experiences, and experience sexuality in a safe and healthy way.

# WHY DO GIRLS HAVE SEX?

This is the real talk about sex. Beyond the talk from your mom or dad, not the talk your friends gave you, but the truth from a real live sex therapist. Half of teens will have sex before they finish high school. Many more girls will have sexual experiences that do not include sexual intercourse, but these sexual encounters are nevertheless important in their lives and affect the way they feel about sex. For most girls, the decision to have sex is a difficult one for a lot of reasons. Most girls want to have sex to have fun and to show love for a person in a special way. Unfortunately, many girls have sex for the wrong reasons, especially sex for the first time. When that happens, many girls have regrets and wish they could turn back the hands of time.

In this chapter, girls talk about why they have sex, with a lot of teens telling their personal stories of the first time they had a sexual experience. Readers need to be cautioned that these stories contain explicit information and details about sexual situations: if you are not ready for this level of sexual detail, this is not the book for you. These real teens share their intimate experiences in order to tell you the truth about having sex as a teenager, so you can use their knowledge to make up your own mind about sex, acquire your own sexual wisdom, and make the best decision for yourself—so that you will have sex for the right reason, when you are ready.

## REASONS GIRLS HAVE SEX

### To Please Their Boyfriends—Jayne's Story

2

> Jayne had her first sexual experience at 15. Her boyfriend "Juan" was 16. He was a "real hottie." Jayne really loved Juan, and therefore she would do anything to make him happy. He wanted to have sex but she didn't. They talked about it and they compromised. Jayne would "take care of" Juan on a regular basis by giving him oral sex. The first time they shared this experience, Jayne was "grossed out" by the act. Mostly, she didn't like Juan coming (or ejaculating semen) in her mouth. She found it unpleasant to say the least, but after a few kisses, a little making out, she would just give him a "blow job." On Friday and Saturday nights, at a minimum, since she wouldn't "put out," she had to give Juan his blow job or she feared he would break up with her and find someone who would "give it up."
>
> Ten years later, Jayne came into therapy, engaged to a new boyfriend and seeking treatment before she got married, because she really didn't want to have sex. When she did engage in sexual acts, in spite of her feelings for her boyfriend, she would cry afterwards.

Having sex to please a boyfriend is a MAJOR reason that teenage girls have sex, even when they don't want to have sex. You need to know that a lot of guys will put pressure on you to have sex if you're going out with them. However, in spite of the fact that some guys don't put any pressure on a girl, some girls still think they HAVE to have sex with their boyfriends because they think that's what a guy wants.

Honestly, it is true, that most teenage guys do want to have sex. For a lot of guys, the urge to have sex is driven by hormones and they can't help but feel this way—they simply want sex. While some girls feel this way to some degree, this urge is usually different than it is for guys. A lot of girls just want to be kissed, hugged, touched, complimented, and loved, but they do not necessarily feel the need to have sex. Conversely, many guys do not feel the same way about sex as girls feel: they are more interested in the physical act of sex first and foremost, considering the emotional, playful closeness that girls like above all else about sex as secondary.

> Remember: Your first and most important obligation in sex, now and forever until you die. . . is to take responsibility for making yourself happy!

You are responsible for making yourself happy, both physically and emotionally. This means that you have to make decisions about sex with which YOU CAN BE HAPPY. This means that YOU are responsible for deciding what you think about sex, for taking into account the feelings you are feeling when you think about sex, and for deciding how you think and feel about your body. You are responsible for deciding how much touching is OK for you or how 'far' you want to go with sexual experiences. Ultimately, many partners do not even know if you are happy or care whether they are doing what *you* want sexually. If you have a really great guy who cares about you, he *will* care if you want to have sex with him. This is great, albeit perhaps rare at an age when young men tend to be ruled by their own needs and driven by their hormones, but a boy cannot read your mind and know what you really want—you have to tell him.

IF you really want to, if *you* feel you are ready to have sex, if *you* are prepared to practice safe sex, AND if *you* want to please the partner you have chosen, THEN sex is your choice. BUT: DO NOT betray your body, mind, or emotions to please someone else. In a later chapter, we will talk about how to *know* if you are really ready for sex.

## In Love—Kayla's Story

Kayla was almost 17 when she fell in love with Tom the summer before their senior year in high school. They were both working at a park, she as a lifeguard and he on the maintenance crew at the golf club. Kayla was attracted to Tom the very first day she met him. He was an all-American athlete, and she was also into sports. The first day they met was a rainy summer day and the whole work crew was hanging out indoors, waiting for the bad weather to pass. Kayla spent a lot of time talking to Tom and found out they had a lot in common. They kissed at work before this first day of their acquaintance had ended. They seemed drawn to each other in a magnetic way, and Kayla and Tom dated very seriously for a month. They saw each other every day during this time and spent many nights sneaking into the park (Tom had a key) to go swimming and skinny dipping and talking under the summer moon. Kissing progressed to touching and loving each other in a special, intimate way. They began to take showers together, play sexually together, and to make love to each other without having sexual intercourse. About mid-summer, Kayla decided Tom was the guy she wanted to make love to for the first time. She was so attracted to him, and they just couldn't keep their hands off of each other. While Tom obviously enjoyed their time together, he had put no pressure on Kayla to have sexual intercourse. He was not a virgin, but he didn't want Kayla to do something she didn't want to do, and he was happy with their sexual relationship the way it was.

Kayla told Tom that she wanted him to be her first. Although she had crushes on guys before, she never felt like having a sexual relationship, beyond touching, with them. Tom and Kayla talked about it a lot. Mostly, Tom wanted to make sure that Kayla was SURE she really wanted to lose her virginity. Kayla decided she was ready. Tom was in charge of getting birth control and the two of them planned out where and when they wanted to have, or could arrange to have, sex.

As it turns out, they first had sex in the back of Tom's car ("he had a car with the backseat the size of a bedroom"), overlooking the water in the park late one night in order to have a lot of privacy. Kayla said they laughed a lot when they first had sex, because she really didn't know what to do—like exactly how to "put it in." Even though Tom had one previous sexual partner, he wasn't very skilled at sex either, and they joked about putting on the condom "the right way." Kayla said that there was a little bit of uncomfortable pressure with his putting his penis inside of her vagina that first time, and she had a little vaginal bleeding, but not a lot. Kayla had a good time and felt even closer to Tom than she had before.

The next time they were together, Tom told her they didn't have to have sex just because they did it before. This made Kayla feel like he really respected her, and, interestingly, made her want to be close to him sexually even more. Their relationship lasted several months, but after a while, probably because they went to different schools and got involved with sports and other friends, they just kind of drifted apart. It wasn't a bad break up, and in fact Kayla said that "it was pretty much mutual." Kayla had no regrets about her first sexual experience.

Several years after her first sexual experience with Tom, Kayla had a positive attitude toward sex. She was in a committed relationship and felt great about guys, too. The guy she was currently with was really sweet, and they were talking about getting married. I think Kayla felt good about men and sexual relationships because she did not have any really horrible early relationships or sexual experiences. Sure, she had some bad times, like being dumped once by a guy she really liked, but she got over it and accepted this loss as a part of life (plus she had great friends to help her through). The important thing is that Kayla was ready for sex, she was in love, and she picked a partner who really respected her. Most importantly: she had no regrets, just a really nice memory of Tom in her heart for many years.

## To Keep Their Boyfriend—Melissa's Story

Melissa was 14, and she really liked Nick, who was 17. She and Nick had been going out for about two months, and they had a lot of fun together, like going to the movies, meeting with friends, walking around the neighborhood, listening to music, and going out to eat. Melissa really enjoyed the time she spent with Nick and they enjoyed hanging out with each other's friends, too. They had kissed, and after a while began to do some big time making out, including touching each other. After only a couple of weeks, Nick began to pressure Melissa to have sex. Melissa was a virgin and she wanted to save sex for when she got married. Nick got mad every time she would stop him from touching her below the waist or from putting her hand on his penis.

Melissa started feeling really uncomfortable about situations when she knew they were going to be alone because Nick would expect her to make out with him. After three months of going out, Nick told her that if she didn't "put out," he was going to break up with her and find someone else who would have sex with him. Melissa really liked Nick and didn't want to lose him, so she finally gave in to him.

Sex hurt Melissa physically and she didn't even like it a little bit. Every time they got together after that, Nick expected to have sex with her, and Melissa would just close her eyes and let him have sex with her while she cried. Nick didn't like it that Melissa wouldn't "get into it," so he broke up with her anyway, after they had been together sexually about seven or eight times.

Melissa wanted me to tell my readers that she really regretted giving in to Nick, that she wished she had never had sex with him. *She did really like him, but she knew she simply wasn't ready for sex. She did it just so he wouldn't break up with her.* As it turns out, they broke up shortly after they had sex anyway, and consequently, she found out that he really didn't care about her feelings, even when she was having sexual intercourse with him. She said it was not "lovemaking," like she imagined first sex would be. It wasn't the great, loving connection that she thought sex would enable her to have with Nick. Because of her choice to have sex with Nick, she stayed away from serious relationships with guys for quite a while after the end of that relationship because she just didn't want to deal with the sexual pressure.

For girls, being dumped because you don't "put out" is a real problem. A lot of guys (and girls) WILL dump you if you don't have sex with them, but the truth is that LOTS of guys will dump you even if you DO have sex with them. BUT: there are a lot of ways to show affection for each other besides having sexual intercourse, which we will discuss later.

Just think: if the guy is not very imaginative with sharing affection and doesn't care enough to do things YOU want to do, do you think you will have much fun sexually with him? You have to decide whether or not this guy is worth it before you actually go all the way with sex. Once again, you have to decide whether or not this is what suits you at this time in your life rather than basing your decision on the expectation of a deepening of the relationship, or the continuation of the relationship at all for that matter, just because you had sex. Melissa found out that Nick did not care enough about her to respect her feelings about sex. Then, as it turned out, when they did have sex, he wasn't concerned (or maybe experienced) enough to be aware of what she wanted in sex or in the relationship, either. So the sexual experience was not only disappointing, but it hurt her, with lingering long-term psychological effects that kept her from having healthy relationships with boys when she was young. Like many young women, she simply avoided boys altogether.

Remember: The question here is, if a guy is not willing to think about your feelings before sex, is he going to think about your feelings during or after sex?

## Curiosity—Jessica's Story

Jessica was 14 when her best friend "Mandy" came to her house for a sleepover. As is typical of sleepovers, they began to talk about guys. They decided they would "practice kissing." This seemed a bit strange to Jessica, but she thought, "What does it matter? I'm just kissing another girl." She thought that this would help her get past the embarrassment of kissing a guy, and Jessica felt very trusting of her friend. She felt that Mandy would never tell anyone about this silly playfulness. What happened, however, was that the practice of kissing kept reoccurring, or kept being "perfected" between the two girls, as Jessica saw it.

Mandy, on the other hand, started being more sexually excited about the situation. Mandy made a move on Jessica and started feeling her breasts. Although Jessica tried to slow things down by pulling Mandy's hands away from her breasts, she did not do so quickly enough to keep Mandy's other hand from sliding down between her legs and touching her genitals. This was shocking and frightening to Jessica. "Wow! Major weirdness!" she thought.

The problem with this situation was not so much that Mandy had feelings of attraction to Jessica, but that Mandy was not honest about her intentions. This incident caused Jessica to feel very weird and uncomfortable around Mandy and it ruined their friendship. Jessica reported that Mandy tried to play off what she did "as a joke," but Jessica knew that Mandy was not joking and had been serious about wanting sexual interaction.

Whether it is a person of the same sex or of the opposite sex, a person who starts sexual interaction has a responsibility to get permission from their partner for physical contact. This includes kissing, but it is particularly important to get permission before touching the breasts or genitals. Also, individuals need to be aware of the kinds of situations they put themselves in that can lead to someone sexually approaching them, whether it is a guy or a girl.

Some girls and guys just have sex because they have heard so much about it, seen so much about it, and thought so much about it that they are dying to find out what it is like. Considering how much our culture shows and talks about sex on TV, in movies, in music videos, and in songs, it is normal to be curious about what sex really *is* like. This is completely natural and understandable.

As a sex therapist who talks to people about their first sexual experiences every week, I will tell you that almost all women and men are disappointed who choose to have sex for the first time only because they are curious.

A lot of the time, if someone is simply curious about sex, it is not the particular person or sexual partner that is important to him or her, but rather, they have sex as a result of simply deciding that they are ready to try it. Consequently, some people, perhaps most, once they have decided they are ready for sex and want to see what it is like are not very choosy when it comes to who their first sexual partner will be. Take a piece of advice: sex feels different when you have loving feelings toward your partner than when you feel nothing emotional toward him or her. In fact, sometimes this difference is as big as the difference between joy and pain, and between emotional and physical pain.

Just having the physical act of a hand touch you, let alone having more intimate physical touching, will not be very fun the first time, most likely, unless there is an emotional component or you have a partner with whom you can talk freely about sex. The first time you have any level of sexual activity, whether it is kissing or touching or something more, can be embarrassing and awkward, so you need to be with a person who knows and understands you. "Just doing it" doesn't lead to very satisfying sex for most people and even if the act feels good physically; it can make you feel bad about yourself emotionally.

## Embarrassed That You Are a Virgin—Tina's Story

> Tina was 20 years old, and she was the only person in her social group who was a virgin. She felt embarrassed that she was a virgin, and one Friday night, she decided to have sex with a friend just to have sex to see what the big deal was. Sex lasted about six minutes. It was painful and there was no pleasure, emotionally or physically. After her first sexual experience, she thought, "Is this all there is? What is the big deal?"

If you are with someone you really don't like that much, or if you're just having sexual intercourse to lose your virginity, you will be missing some of the "specialness" of sex, including the emotional satisfaction, emotional connection, and physical bonding that can make for a wonderful experience. An emotional connection means finding a person with whom you can talk, someone with whom you feel comfortable outside of a sexual situation and who treats you right. Girls who are virgins, especially if they are planning to have first sexual experiences, need to be with someone who is sensitive to their inexperience and emotional vulnerability. Also, virgins need to take sex for the first time much, much more slowly physically than six minutes, to avoid physical pain. Chapter 9 will discuss and explain about sex for the first time, without physical or emotional pain. Again, there is a very different feeling when one has a sexual experience that is combined with a loving connection. For Tina, that connection simply wasn't there, and consequently, it wasn't until much later in her life, when she experienced "lovemaking" as opposed to simply experiencing sex, that she figured out "what the big deal was."

Wait to be with someone who really cares about you, period. It will be worth the wait!

## To Lose Their Virginity Like They Think Their Friends Have—Janice and Anna's Story

Janice didn't like sex and decided she didn't like men either, including her husband. At 32, Janice came in for sex therapy because she didn't want to have sex anymore, and she actually said she simply did not like men. Janice had divorced her husband six months earlier because he had an affair with a co-worker. Janice blamed herself for his cheating because she did not have sex with her husband very often. She was depressed, sad, had no interest in anything, and finally came into therapy.

When discussing her past, it was uncovered that Janice was raped by her mother's boyfriend at age 13. Rape is when someone forces you to have sex (see Chapter 10 on rape). Janice was told by the boyfriend that, if she told anyone, he would tell her father that her mother was a whore and had boyfriends in and out of the apartment all of the time so that her father would get custody of Janice. Janice did not want her father to have custody of her, and she didn't want to move out of her neighborhood, where she had the same friends since first grade. So she never told anyone about the rape. After seeing the rapist's ugliness, and the ugliness in her own father during her parent's divorce, she simply decided she did not like men.

Even Janice's own mother didn't really like men. Janice's father had abandoned the family, supposedly leaving for another woman, and he had left Janice's mother and the two children in poverty. Janice grew up hard. Her mother dated a few men, but she never remarried.

Janice got married because, when her husband asked her to marry him, she thought it would be her only chance at having marriage and a family. Janice was overweight and did not think of herself as very attractive, and she thought that his love for her would be enough to sustain her. Janice didn't really fall in love with her husband, and in fact she didn't think that she could love any man.

After Janice was raped, she still considered herself a virgin technically, and she felt embarrassed about that fact by the time she was 16. When she was a junior in high school, she had sex with the town "bad boy," who had sex with anyone and everyone, just so she wouldn't feel "stupid" about being a virgin because she thought all her friends were having sex. The sex with the "bad boy" was physically painful and emotionless, and right then and there, she decided that she hated sex. Janice never talked to the boy again. She had sex for the wrong reason, with the wrong person, and, as she summed it up, the whole experience "done her wrong." Janice said she felt like a "switch" turned off *that day* and she was no longer interested in sex, nor in trusting or loving men.

Twenty years ago, it was embarrassing for anyone to know you were not a virgin. Now, in some parts of the country, it is equally embarrassing for anyone to know that you are a virgin. So, in some cases, girls want to have sex so that they will not be virgins, because they do not want to feel uncomfortable with being sexually inexperienced, assuming that all their friends are experienced.

"Like they think all their friends are . . . " Let me tell you, not every one of your friends who says they have or have not had sex is telling you the truth. Remember, only half of teens have had sex before they finish high school, which leaves a lot of girls who are still virgins at 17 or 18, and many are still virgins into their 20s. Also, 90% of girls who have sex before 16 regret their first sexual experiences. Waiting until you are ready, waiting for the right sexual partner, waiting until you are in love, and for some women waiting until you are married, is the right decision. Chapter 4 talks about how to know if you're ready to have sex, and what kinds of things you need to think about before sex. If you wait until at least you think you are ready, you will be less likely to regret sexual experiences and hate sex.

Anna came from a religiously conservative family. She was rebellious with her parents and began to hang out with "fast friends," meaning they were drinking, smoking weed and a lot of them were having sex by the time she was in 9th grade. When Anna started hanging out with this group, a lot of people in the high school thought that she, too, was sexually active and promiscuous, which means having sex with a lot of different partners. To feel comfortable with her friends, she told them that she had indeed had sex with lots of different guys. The truth was, however, she was a virgin until 11th grade. By 11th grade, she began to feel scared that everyone would figure out that she was lying, and she also wanted to know if someone wanted her sexually.

So one day, on a first date with a guy she thought only asked her out for sex anyway, she got really drunk because she really wasn't ready for sex. She went with him to an old abandoned, "skanky" barn filled with rats and gave in to his sexual advances. She lost her virginity to a guy she hardly knew and didn't even like. To make matters worse, after sex, she was lying on the ground and he just got up and left her there! She had to walk a long way home because she couldn't tell her parents about where she was or what had happened.

By this time, she couldn't share with her friends that she had sex for the first time because they all thought she had been sexually active for a couple of years. Privately, she felt really alone, stupid, and guilty. She never heard from that guy after their only date, and on top of that she began to drink heavily to drown her feelings of guilt and depression and became an alcoholic. A few months later, she was babysitting and she began to drink heavily from the parents' liquor cabinet. She vomited and passed out in the middle of their family room. When the parents came home, they called her parents and called an ambulance. She went to the hospital for alcohol poisoning. Anna was very embarrassed about the babysitting situation, and her parents were horrified by her behavior. She was punished severely, but she never got any counseling or other help for her problems.

Sadly, Anna came in for counseling because she was not interested in sex. Also, she had gained a lot of weight during her seven-year marriage. Although she had mostly given up alcohol, she had since turned to food for comfort and emotional security. It took a long time for Anna to learn to "reclaim her own sexuality" and to want to have sex with her husband because she wanted to have sex rather than just to fulfill her husband's needs.

## Intoxicated—Mercedes' Story

Mercedes was 14. She came in for therapy because she had had an unwanted sexual experience and couldn't talk to her parents about it. Her father worked in another town, and he wasn't around much to give her any attention. Mercedes' mother was really nice and talked to her about almost anything, but when it came to boys, she didn't even want Mercedes to KISS a guy, let alone to go any further. Mercedes had an older sister, "Dana," who had everything and got most of her mother's attention. Dana was a great student, was on student council, and was even the Homecoming Queen. Mercedes, while she was beautiful, was the opposite of her sister. She had Attention Deficit Disorder, no interest in school, and got in trouble a lot for getting bad grades.

Mercedes looked outside of the house for fun and attention. Sometimes, she had trouble getting close to people because she did not have much confidence in herself. Even in small groups of people, she didn't talk much, and she sat on the sidelines smiling. She had learned to laugh at the right times, like she did in her own family, rather than sharing her opinion because she was used to being criticized. After all, she was the "spacey" one, not the "smart one."

Mercedes started drinking at 13—just a couple of beers here and there. Then she tried marijuana. Mercedes liked smoking weed with friends, because then everyone else was spacey, just like she supposedly was naturally. Mercedes was flirtatious and she liked the attention from guys. She was really pretty and built like a Victoria's Secret model in the 9th grade, so the attention was inevitable. One night, partying at a friend's house, a friend whose parents weren't home, she met a guy who was very nice to her, gave her a lot of compliments and made her feel good about herself. She was drunk and high, which lowered her sexual inhibitions, and she was not experienced at speaking up for herself. She ended up having sexual intercourse for the first time with this guy that she didn't even know. She felt very guilty for having sex.

15

Her family values were against having sex until you were at least much older and in a serious relationship with someone you loved or when you are were married. The sex hurt her physically too, and she had no pleasure after the first five minutes of kissing and touching.

Mercedes cried half of the first session I saw her, and remember, she is only 14 and talking about her first sexual experience: "Things . . . went . . . too far . . . too fast." Mercedes cried for the fact that she couldn't take it back. All she thought about now was how stupid she was . . . like her family made her feel about herself anyway. She now felt more distant from her family than ever. To make it worse, months later, her "virginal" smart sister found out about her sexual encounter and told her dad. Dana said that she was genuinely worried about her sister, which may be true, but Mercedes did not buy that. The whole family talked to her about the incident and repeatedly expressed how disappointed they were in her, especially since the guy was not even a "real boyfriend" and basically "she had engaged in casual sex," which was horrifying to her mother. Dana felt badly for Mercedes, but she felt justified in her betrayal because she was "saving her younger sister."

Even two weeks after the family confrontation between Mercedes and her sister, mother and father, which basically emphasized what a "whore" she had been, she felt very depressed and distant from her family. That is when she came in for therapy.

First, Mercedes needed help not only because she was depressed and was even having thoughts of suicide, but because she also needed to know that she was a good person, and not a loser like her family thought. Second, she needed support in talking about making a mistake sexually. Third, Mercedes had to seriously examine her use of alcohol and drugs and how it affected her judgment and behavior. Mercedes decided to stop using alcohol after that.

Mercedes also needed to know that she wasn't a whore because she had sex, like her family told her she was, even if it was a mistake. Having sex is not a choice between being a virgin or a whore. Even though Mercedes had a bad sexual experience and she wished it did not happen, she did not want to feel guilty, depressed or bad about herself if she chose to have a sexual relationship with someone she truly cared for in the future. Healthy sex and healthy choices include a third option other than to *be a virgin or be a whore*. This third option is that you can be sexually active and not be a bad person, but you have to make responsible decisions that are absolutely right for you.

Certainly, you have read about the effects of alcohol and drugs on sexual inhibitions. Inhibition in this context refers to how much control you have in terms of doing what you want to do or feeling comfortable if you decide to say no to sex. It is absolutely true that drugs and alcohol affect your feelings about sexual decisions. Any reasons that you personally have about wanting or not wanting to have sex suddenly seem less important when you are under the influence of drugs or alcohol. It is very easy to let go of, or even to forget, your important values about sex, to be overtaken by the excitement of the moment and the feeling of being with someone when you are high or drunk. Even your sexual feelings or sexual desire may be intensified when on drugs or alcohol.

It is very easy to feel that having sex in the heat of the moment is OK when you are high, tipsy or drunk, whether you are a virgin or not. Unfortunately, many times in this situation, you will not feel OK the next day or when you are not high or drunk, and the only time to make a decision about sex with a person is when you are not drunk or high. You also need to examine your feelings about having had sex when you are sober. That is when your true feelings will let you make the best decision, without the mind-altering effects of drugs or alcohol.

You also must be aware that there are "date-rape drugs." Three drugs are most commonly used: Rohypol or "roofies," GHB, and Ketamine, which will be discussed in Chapter 10. Other drugs can also be used on unsuspecting victims, such as LSD or tranquilizers.

Drugs can be put in a drink, even a soft drink, like a Coke or juice, without your knowledge, and this can enable an unscrupulous person to take advantage of you.

> You should never let anyone else make a drink for a you, even if you think you know them!

If you begin to feel very drowsy or intoxicated for little or no reason (that is, you haven't had that much of anything to drink or any other drugs), then go to your friends immediately and ask for help. If you have to leave the place where you find yourself in this condition, go to a neighbor's house or apartment, or to a public place and call the police. Call 911 from where you are if possible and get out of there. Some drugs are very fast acting. For further information on drugs, sex, and date rape, read Chapter Ten.

## To Be Sexually Experienced—Rayleen's Story

Rayleen was a freshman in college. She wanted to go home for Christmas to see her high school sweetie, but she was embarrassed that she was still a virgin and she didn't want to be sexually inexperienced with her boyfriend. Rayleen was very religious, which had made sex out of the question in high school. During her freshman year at college, she met a seemingly very sincere, sensitive, and attentive Christian young man, "Marcus." Rayleen made it clear to Marcus that she was in love with a guy from high school, but she dated Marcus anyway.

Rayleen told Marcus that she did not want to go home a virgin, and she and Marcus made a date specifically to have intercourse, which would be the beginning and the end of their sexual relationship. Rayleen had sex with Marcus just to figure out "how to have sex." A few days later, Rayleen went home for Christmas and hooked up with her true love. After Christmas break, Rayleen returned to campus with her new "fiancé" and introduced him to Marcus as her friend. The high school boyfriend never knew about Marcus and Rayleen having sex.

Rayleen never actually revealed her feelings to Marcus, which were that she wanted to ultimately feel in control of both men, because she felt like she wanted to have power over her own sexuality. She thought she would feel better about having sex with her boyfriend if she wasn't a virgin, but as it turned out, instead of feeling in control, she felt like she lost the "specialness" of sharing her virginity with the man she really loved.

Everyone is sexually inexperienced when they are a virgin, and that is how it is expected to be. It is not a federal crime. It can be very sweet and endearing (and fun!) to explore your sexuality with someone loving and understanding of your sexual inexperience. Actually, some people are very inexperienced and unsure of themselves with sex, even if they have had multiple sexual experiences. For one thing, everyone is different when it comes to sexual likes and dislikes. Every couple needs fresh, new exploration with each other in order to discover their own special way of making love together as the relationship evolves. Even couples who have been together for years find that a single sexual encounter can involve discovering something new about their lover, what that one person wants on that one particular day. In fact, sexuality is something that can continue to be new and different over the course of your entire life. It is much more fulfilling to explore this with someone special, with someone to whom you are attracted, with whom you are in love.

## Opportunity of the 'Best' Partner—Jon's Story

Jon came in for sex therapy when he was 18. He had tried to have sex three times with this beautiful girl, "Amber," but he couldn't. Jon thought Amber was just the hottest girl at school, but he really didn't have any feelings for her emotionally. When he finally got his chance to be with her, he couldn't get an erection! In his words, Jon whispered to me, embarrassed, "No matter what I did, my dick just wouldn't get hard!" First, Jon thought about going to get Viagra (a prescription drug generally for older men who have problems with erections), but he decided to talk to a sex therapist instead.

Jon was talking to a lot of girls and was dating a girl other than "Amber," although they weren't in an exclusive relationship. When he was having sex with his girlfriend, Jon didn't have any problems, but Jon was very worried because he really found "Amber" to be so beautiful: she had one of the hottest bodies he had ever seen. He really was excited to be with her and more excited when she asked him to have sex with her. Amber was 17 and was a virgin. She wanted to give her virginity to Jon. She didn't even care for Jon that much; she just felt that she was not only ready for sex but wanted to lose her virginity, to try sex, with him. Jon couldn't have been more excited, but when it came to actually having sexual intercourse, Jon just couldn't "get it up." He just didn't understand what was wrong with him and he was worried about his performance and his reputation.

Sex is more than just the functions of the body. Every person has his or her own "conditions for sex." For some people, that means being married. For some people, that means being in love. For others, it is having an available sexual partner to whom they are attracted in some way. For Jon, finding out that he really didn't like Amber that much was sufficient to put a damper on his physical desire for her. That is, he found her physically beautiful, but he didn't have any loving feelings for her. When it came down to it, he felt guilty about "making love" and "taking her virginity" when he knew he wasn't in love with her or wasn't "the one" for whom she was looking, and he couldn't do it.

Jon found out the hard way (or soft way) that one of his "conditions" for enjoying sex was that he had to have emotional feelings for someone and he couldn't just be satisfying someone else, or satisfying his own physical urges for that matter. Jon felt really badly about himself at first, because he saw himself as this big sexual stud-muffin who could do anything, anytime, any way to please someone, but he couldn't. He was a human being with human emotions. Jon learned to respect that about himself, to respect the "wisdom of his penis," as it were, and learn his conditions for lovemaking. Chapter 4 talks more about recognizing your own "conditions" for sex. Jon also realized he should respect his body and not even THINK of taking Viagra (a drug to give men erections) to overrule his body's emotions.

Jon's story, even though it is a story from a guy, is included in this chapter, so girls will know that not all guys are just after sex from girls. Some guys are sensitive, caring, compassionate and have emotional reasons, and conditions, for having sex. Not all guys are just driven by hormones, as girls are often told, and "after one thing—sex." Some guys really are interested and driven by emotions, too.

## Anger and Competition—Gwen's Story

Gwen was a sophomore in college. She was a virgin and sexually inexperienced. Gwen had a best friend, Mackie, with whom she talked about everything. Gwen wanted to experience sex, like Mackie, and to be able to talk to her about sexual experiences. Mackie began to spend more and more time with her own boyfriend instead of with Gwen. One night, Gwen was fixing a special dinner for her and Mackie, but Mackie blew her off to spend time with her boyfriend. Gwen felt incredibly insecure, worthless and angry.

Gwen went out and found a party on campus, which was primarily made up of college athletes. Although there were other girls at the party who tried to warn her about guys at the party, who told her NOT to take guys home, Gwen became angry and defiant. Gwen was mad at Mackie, and she felt very alone. She got very drunk and invited numerous guys back to her dorm room.

The next thing that Gwen remembers was being in a dorm room

and the guys were taking turns having sexual intercourse with her. About 20 different guys, most of them from the football team, had sex with her that night. Gwen consented to having sexual relations with these men, so it was not technically rape, but the consent was based upon her feelings of hurt about Mackie and her sense of competition with Mackie and her boyfriend and the fact that she was quite drunk. Gwen felt like, if she had sexual experiences, she could regain her friendship with Mackie and not feel like a sexual social outcast. Unfortunately, Gwen became emotionally disturbed by the sexual episode in the dorm room. She never maintained a stable relationship with a man after that incident.

Although Gwen was highly intelligent and successful in her career, she felt like she was "dirty." She never had children because she felt she was "a bad person" and would make a bad mother. She never did keep her friendship with Mackie, who found out about what happened, as did a lot of other people, and Gwen was ultimately rejected by her friends. Although Gwen was quite smart, just finishing college was very hard for her.

Gwen came in for therapy much later in life, when she was 42 years old. She was depressed. Gwen still thought about that night with the football team, and she thought about it at least every week of her life if not more often. One of the things that made the situation so bad was that Gwen would continually run into one of the guys involved and jokes would be made about that night. Even at football games at her old college, 10 years later, it always seemed like she would run into someone who would make a joke about her. Gwen had very low self-esteem, and she still thought of herself as "just a big slut."

Gwen avoided dating for a long time, even though she was very attractive and was asked out a lot. She didn't get serious with a guy until she was 37, and when she later married Gwen didn't have a good sexual relationship with her husband because she still felt angry toward men and sex.

## Anger at Parents/Absent Parents—Lauren's Story

Lauren was raised in an extremely fundamentalist religious family, which can be best described as very conservative in their sexual views. Her family very rarely talked about relationships and never talked about sexual relationships. At Lauren's church youth fellowship, there were opportunities to meet guys who went to the church, but only under the direct supervision of church adults.

The summer of Lauren's 14th year was like other summers in her life: she went to church camp. However, that summer was different because as a camp counselor, she was given a great deal more freedom. For the first time, Lauren found herself able to meet a nice guy and get to know him without the heavy supervision that she had experienced most of her life whenever she was with a boy. Lauren had deeply resented this interference and felt angry toward her parents for giving her no freedom in her life at home. However, without them around, she was lost when it came to how to talk to a guy or handle herself alone with him.

The summer started with the excitement of meeting a guy she liked and who liked her in return. Because of the clear guilt and shameful teachings regarding sex she had received in the church to which her family belonged, any behaviors that would lead to sex were clearly forbidden. After two weeks at camp, however, things had gone pretty far with this guy, with kissing and touching that stopped just short of oral sex and intercourse. When she was with the guy, she was also thinking about the anger she felt toward her parents, but she was convinced that her actions reflected her newfound freedom. Later, however, after an interaction with the guy, she always regretted what she had done and felt ashamed.

Years later, by the time Lauren came to her first therapy session, she had been married for five years and was headed toward divorce. She didn't have any sexual feelings, and her husband could no longer accept her excuses for not having sex. Ever since her first

**sexual contact that summer at the age of 14, she had always felt that sex was wrong somehow; and actually having sex seemed to make her feel that she was a bad person.**

Even though Lauren didn't have sexual intercourse at 14, and even though she stayed a virgin until she was married, she had a lot of distress about sex and relationships. Mostly, Lauren was not prepared for relationships with men, due in a large part to the excessive emotional control of her church and her family. Lauren never got to experience friendships with guys, dating, or even talking about relationships because of the restrictions in her religious order. By the time she had the opportunity to even talk to a guy freely, she didn't really know what to do and made a mistake by doing things for which she would later feel guilty. In fact, what she did end up doing made her feel so guilty that she didn't date until she was much older. When she got married, she was still unprepared for interacting with a man, especially sexually. Through the process of therapy, Lauren was able to talk about her deep feelings of guilt and shame, and ultimately she began to live a normal life and gave her marriage a new start. For further discussion on religion and sexuality, read Jennifer's story, in Chapter 2. Note that not all religions may cause this type of scary guilt, and many religious leaders are open to discussions and providing guidance to teenagers on sexuality; unfortunately, this was Lauren's true story and experience with religion and massive guilt.

## To Be Loved—Suzanna's Story

**Suzanna was the only child in a single-parent family. This in itself was not a problem, except in her case, at the age of 12, Suzanna acted as the adult and watched over her mother who had a severe drinking problem. Suzanna's father married six weeks after her parents divorced, had two other children in two years, and for whatever**

reasons of his own, had nothing to do with her. Suzanna wanted so much to be really loved and liked by others. When she was in middle school, most of her friends were older high school boys who gave her the attention that she thought she wanted and needed.

Things progressed very quickly for her with these guys because they were very experienced with sex and Suzanna confused sex with love. She also depended on the guys to take care of her and to know how sex was supposed to happen. As a result, Suzanna ended up having four different sexual partners before she was 14 years old. She reported that she would just put her hands over her face and these boys would do the rest. Suzanna got pregnant, dropped out of high school, and got married to one of the guys at 15; he was 18. She had her second child when she was 17.

Suzanna came in for therapy at this point in her life, when she was 17, married, and the mother of two children. She felt like she was trapped, stuck in her life. She was gaining weight, and she felt depressed. In therapy, she realized that sex was not physically, emotionally or psychologically satisfying, and that she was just looking for love. In short, she realized that she had confused sex for love. She even thought that, if she got pregnant, at least she would have someone to love or the guy would love her more and have to stay around because of the baby. Fortunately, Suzanna did feel like she got a little lucky, because her husband loved her and she loved him, which was good. Unfortunately, she felt like she missed really growing up and being her own person. At 17, she had to start to figure out what she wanted in life, which was not easy with two very young children to raise.

Do not confuse sex with love!

## Natural Interest—Brittany's Story

Brittany was 14 when she first had sex. She was at camp. She had gone to the same camp for several years, and she loved the place and the people. Often, she and her friends would ogle at the guys at the coed camp and plot ways to sneak out in the night to meet with them. Brittany was an early bloomer with a great body, and she got a lot of attention from the older guys. She had a huge crush on "Chad." She and Chad talked for weeks and were considered to be going together by all bystanders. Brittany wanted to have sex. She was curious and she thought that she was ready for sex. She and Chad talked about the prospect and planned out how they could accomplish it. He got the condoms, and she figured out a way to sneak out. He was a 17 year-old junior camp counselor. She describes her first sexual experience as "slightly painful, but exciting," and she said she had no regrets.

Devastatingly, Chad never talked to her again after they had sex. Immediately after their midnight meeting, he avoided her, ignored her, and began to pay attention to other girls. Brittany felt enormously betrayed and hurt by the fact that she had shared herself sexually only to be rejected.

After that summer, Brittany made a decision that sex was meaningless and to never attach emotions to sex. She became quite promiscuous, having sexual intercourse with at least 75 different partners before she graduated from college. She met a really nice guy in her senior year of college, with whom she fell in love and married. Unfortunately, after two years of marriage, she felt no sexual desire for him and came in for counseling.

Brittany learned to attach no meaning to sex and no emotions to it either. So even when she wanted to have emotions connected to sex, she couldn't manage it. When Brittany had sex for the first time, she had a natural interest in sex. She was really attracted to her boyfriend, and she was interested in and wanted to have sex. She also felt quite strongly that she was ready for sex, emotionally and biologically, and she prepared herself for protection from pregnancy and diseases. Unfortunately, she was very hurt by sex, because of the way her boyfriend treated her after they were together. Sometimes, even if you think you and your partner are ready for sex, it is important to know you can trust your partner so that you won't get hurt later by the relationship. Later in this book, I talk about ways to avoid getting hurt emotionally by sex, particularly by knowing how you can trust a guy not to use you sexually.

## Momentary Passion—Morgan's Story

Morgan was 17 and was spending the weekend with her girlfriend, at her girlfriend's parent's beach house. It was the summer, and there were a lot of teenagers at the beach at that time. Morgan met a guy at the pier one day, when she and her friends went there to hear a band that was playing. It was a common hangout area for teens. The next day, Morgan and her friends met "Daniel" at the beach for a swim. The whole day was a blast for everyone. The whole group, Morgan and her friends and Daniel and his friends, swam, ate, sunbathed, played volleyball, and just walked around. Everyone laughed and had a great time.

That night, Morgan planned to meet Daniel for a midnight walk on the beach. It was a hot, moonlit night. They kissed and touched each other. They decided to go skinny-dipping for fun. They both stripped down to their underwear and hit the waves at high tide. Daniel kept on playfully grabbing at Morgan, and she liked it. She did not know Daniel very well, but she was having fun. She began to get turned on by his touching and was playfully touching him, too. They fell into the waves together, kissed, and laughed some more. Eventually, they completely undressed, throwing their underclothes onto the beach. Morgan told Daniel she did not want to go all the way, and he said OK.

The two of them ended up making out on the sand dunes together. They were passionate together and got caught up in the moment of passion under the stars of a summer's night. Daniel did not pressure her, but Morgan was very sexually excited and wanted to have sex. They didn't use any birth control or even a condom. It was a wonderful moment, but the next day, Morgan realized that she had been merely caught up in the moment and perhaps she had made a mistake in going all the way with Daniel.

Morgan never saw Daniel or his friends again. He called her the next day, but after that, she returned home, and she never heard from him again, even though they had exchanged phone numbers. While it was a fun, passionate moment, Morgan always thought she would have sex for the first time with someone she loved. She hadn't used birth control and she was worried about being pregnant every day for three weeks until her period finally did come. She didn't even know Daniel's last name, and she thought if she had gotten pregnant, she really didn't even know who the father was! She did ask Daniel if he had any sexually transmitted diseases, and he said he didn't. But since she didn't know him, she really didn't know if he was telling the truth, and she ended up making her first trip to a gynecologist to get tested for sexually transmitted diseases, which she found embarrassing.

Often girls have sex because they are swept away in the moment. Perhaps a girl is with someone she really cares about, but maybe sex is not even on her mind. However, in a moment of passion, with deep kissing and touching, people get turned on and it's difficult to turn off those immense feelings. While the moment was passionate and positive for Morgan, she was not sexually responsible and she paid the price for it in her worry about pregnancy alone. She was lucky: she did not get pregnant or catch any diseases, but she had to go through a scare (and take a trip to the doctor) to pay the price for an hour's worth of passion.

## Special Occasion—Georgia's Story

It was the 1960s, and Georgia was 19 and had been going out with Terry, who was 21, for two years. Terry was drafted to go to the Vietnam War. Being drafted meant you had to fight in the war; you didn't have a choice. Georgia and Terry had talked about getting married, but Georgia was not sure that Terry was the guy for her, because he seemed to have a lot of family problems. Terry and Georgia had gotten into a lot of fights, and they had broken up twice, but when he was just about to be sent to Vietnam, they were still together. Georgia thought that there was a good chance that Terry would never make it back from Vietnam, because a lot of young men died in that war. After he was drafted, Georgia lived in Florida and Terry was stationed in the Army in California. She took a five-day bus trip all the way out to California to see Terry off to war. Because she was afraid she would never see him again, she decided to have sex with him. They had played a lot together sexually before, but they never "went all the way."

Secretly, Georgia wished Terry would die in Vietnam. She felt really awful for saying this, but Terry had been very possessive, very pushy, constantly harassed her for sex, and she was not assertive enough to just say no to him. So, when Georgia had sex for the first time, she did it just because it was a special occasion. She did not have sex because she wanted to, but because she felt sorry for Terry having to go to war, guilty for her thoughts about his death, and because she wanted him to have a good memory from home before he left for war.

As it turned out, Georgia got pregnant! She had to tell her Catholic mother—and being pregnant and unmarried was considered a terrible thing in 1960. And in 1960, almost always, when you got pregnant, you got married. So, Georgia felt like she had to get married to Terry, which they did when he had one leave home from his two years of overseas duty. Not only did Georgia have to go through a pregnancy by herself, but she had to take care of the baby all by herself for two years. She also had to live with her parents, and all because she felt sorry for Terry and it was a special occasion.

Partly because of her Catholic religion, and partly because Terry was the father of her children, Georgia stayed with Terry for 35 years. They had four children together. In spite of the years and the children they raised together, however, they never had a good marriage: Terry came back from Vietnam addicted to drugs and with more mental problems than he had when he left. For many years, it was just Georgia and her kids, and Terry did whatever he wanted to do, even showing up only when he felt like it. Georgia deeply regretted her trip to California for many years. She deeply regretted giving in to sex just because Terry was going to war. Mostly, she made the best of it, but it took 35 years and her children leaving home before she decided to make decisions for herself and to start doing what she wanted.

Georgia wanted to tell this story to help other girls, and to give girls two messages: 1. Get out of a relationship if it is not right. Speak up for yourself. If you fight *all* the time *before* marriage, it will only get worse, and, 2. Never have sex because you are pressured to do it, even if it is a special occasion. If it is right, there will be plenty of time when it is right for *both* of you.

## To Hurt Another Guy—Maria's Story

Maria liked Carlos, and she was extremely jealous that Carlos was having sex with Theresa. To hurt Carlos, she went out with another guy, a white guy at their largely Hispanic school. Maria had sex with the other guy, "in every which way, six ways to sundown," just to get Carlos' attention. Maria then told Carlos' best friend, "Tex," whom she knew would tell Carlos in detail what she had done. Maria thought that having sex with Pete would make Carlos jealous, and moreover, that it would make him want her. Actually, the plan worked, and Carlos did hook up with Maria. But, after having sex with Carlos, Maria dumped him like a bad habit.

Girls and guys can get used in relationships and for sex. People of all ethnicities—white, Black, Hispanic, and others—can learn to use sex as a game and use it to hurt other people. Using sex as a weapon is a trick as old as time, so both girls and guys need to watch out for this and to learn how to prevent it from happening to them. People can play a lot of games. For most people, a sexual relationship is more important than just a game. Most people want sharing intimacy to be special, but for some it isn't necessary to be loved or to love to have sex with another person. Make sure you are treated special: You deserve it.

## To See If You're Gay—Zoe's Story

Zoe was 21 and in college. She was dating a guy named "Kyle." Zoe really liked Kyle a lot and they had had a sexual relationship for several months. She was happy with him and had a lot of fun with him, including their sexual relationship. They'd even talked about getting married after they graduated from college. Zoe had been sexually active since she was 17, and she had mostly positive sexual relationships with guys. Zoe was taking a Women's Studies class in college, which included subjects such as feminism, women's rights, and lesbian rights. It was the summer term in college and Zoe had stayed on campus to take an extra class, as well as to be on her own, away from her family. Kyle was living at home, in another town, working, and he and Zoe only saw each other about every other weekend. Zoe was pretty sure she was "straight" because she was attracted to guys, but thinking about gay rights and all of the other heady ideas to which she was being exposed made her wonder if she would like sex with a woman. She was pretty experimental with heterosexual sex, and she didn't want to go through life, get married, and later find out she liked sex more with women and that she'd missed something all those years.

"Zoe" met another woman, "Frannie," in her summer class. They had lunch a few times and talked about how you know if you're gay or straight. Frannie had also only been with men and thought she was straight, too. Frannie and Zoe became friends. The subject of how to know if you're gay kept coming up, maybe because of the class they were in, but maybe there was some attraction between them as well. Also, Zoe felt sexually lonely without her boyfriend in town most of the summer. The two of them decided to try to have sex together and see if they liked it. Zoe felt like sex with Frannie was "kinda flat," and that it wasn't that exciting. In fact, she didn't even like the idea of giving a woman oral sex: for her, it was a real turn off just to think about it. As friends, however, they both got to experience sex with a woman. It was interesting for both of them and kind of sweet between friends. Zoe was glad she had the experience, but she decided it just wasn't for her. She was glad that she just knew who she was sexually and understood the experience to be harmless sexual experimentation.

For Zoe, experimenting sexually with a woman was a good thing for her to do. Even though she didn't like it, it wasn't a bad experience. Sexual curiosity of sexual orientation is common for people. In Chapter 3, we will talk about how to know if you're gay and what to do about it.

# two

# WHY DON'T GIRLS
# WANT TO HAVE SEX?

It is a myth that all teenagers want to have sex. The top four reasons girls don't want to have sex are: religious and moral reasons, fear of pregnancy, "haven't found the right partner," and the fear of STDs. Yes, girls delay sex for a lot of personal reasons, and important reasons, some of which are included in this chapter. No, not everyone is having sex, and here are the numbers to prove it!

## Age and Race of First Intercourse

| All Teen Girls | Any Sexual Contact | Sexual Intercourse | Oral Sex |
|---|---|---|---|
| Age 15 | 34% | 26% | 26% |
| Age 16 | 50% | 40% | 42% |
| Age 17 | 64% | 49% | 56% |
| Age 18 | 78% | 70% | 70% |
| Age 19 | 88% | 77% | 74% |
| **Ages 15–19** | | | |
| Hispanic | 59% | 49% | 47% |
| White | 64% | 52% | 58% |
| Black | 68% | 62% | 53% |

(National Center for Health Statistics, 2005)

As you can see, the older girls get, the more likely they are to have sexual experiences, including oral sex and sexual intercourse. Interestingly, sexual experiences vary depending on one's ethnicity or race. For example, black girls are more likely to experience sexual intercourse at an early age, but white girls are more likely to give or receive oral sex. Hispanic or Latino girls are less likely to engage in any type of sexual activity, delaying sexual experiences until later in life (National Center for Health Statistics, 2005).

## REASONS GIRLS AREN'T READY FOR SEX

### Simply Not Ready—Shawana's Story

Shawana was 14 and in 9th grade. She was talking to and spending time with Dwayne, who was 17 and a senior in high school. One night, she met Dwayne at the movies. He kissed her and tried to touch her breasts. Shawana moved his hand away from her breasts, telling him, "No." Dwayne kept calling her, but Shawana decided to stop talking to him. Shawana had heard that Dwayne had had sex with a few other girls and that he wanted to have sex with her, too. Shawana was very inexperienced in having relationships: she had only had a boyfriend once for three weeks, and all they did was kiss. Shawana decided she was not ready for the pressure of sex in a relationship. She figured that if Dwayne was trying to touch her sexually, on her breasts, on their first "date" there was no way she was ready for more of a relationship with him, so she broke off the relationship.

For the right reasons or the wrong reasons, some people are not ready for sex. For most girls and women, they just know what is right in their heart or in their gut. They may not be ready for any of the reasons discussed below, or they may not be ready for other reasons, or the reasons may be unknown, buried within the girl's psyche. The fact remains that many girls and women REALLY DO know when they are ready for sexual exploration, whether that is kissing or big time making out or oral sex or sexual intercourse.

Many people ask me this question: "How do I know if I am ready for sex?" In Chapter 4, we will discuss at length how to know if you are ready for sex. But I will tell you that MOST girls know when they are *not* ready for sex, because they simply are not ready. This is one of the best reasons for NOT having sex, because somewhere in your body, heart or your soul, not for any reason that you can really figure out, you are not ready. This can be true when you are a virgin, and it can be true when you are sexually experienced. It can be true when you are young or 80 years old. It is very important that you listen to and respect this feeling or thought, or you will feel like you are betraying yourself. Do what your heart and mind are urging you to do.

Do not have sex until you are ready!

## Religious Training—Jennifer's Story

Jennifer had her first sexual experience at 13. Jennifer's father was an alcoholic. He went to work before she got up for school and returned home when she was in bed or going to bed. When he was home, everyone was afraid of him, as he frequently had alcoholic fits of anger. Jennifer had a good relationship with her mom, but her mom was busy taking care of two younger kids, doing ALL the housework, and keeping up with the family's social life on the weekends. Jennifer was scared in her own house. She felt like she was unimportant to her family, and she wanted to get out of her house as much as possible.

Then she met Peter. Peter was 15 or 16. He was interesting. He went to church. The youth group did fun things, so Jennifer joined. She started having a lot of fun and keeping active a couple of nights a week and most of the time during weekends. Since it was church stuff that she was involved in, her dad agreed to most of the activities. Jennifer really liked Peter a lot and loved the attention he gave her and the fun they had together. Then Peter wanted sex. Jennifer didn't want it, but she felt like she had to say yes or she would lose Peter as a boyfriend. After all, girls his age were "all having sex" and he could have "anyone he wanted." Jennifer felt like she had to have sex or she would lose out on all the attention and all the fun she had discovered with Peter, and furthermore she wouldn't be able to get out of the house, which was perhaps her highest priority. So she said no, and said no, and said no to Peter because she didn't want to have sex. Then, fearful of rejection, she didn't say no.

In fact, Jennifer really didn't say yes, but she didn't say no either. The first sexual experience was sudden, surprising, painful, did not provide any pleasure to her, and was over very quickly. Afterwards, she felt very guilty. Her guilt was partly because she felt that having premarital sex was wrong for religious reasons and partly because she was told by her parents not to have sex until she was married. Jennifer felt guilty for months, and then months turned into years. She stayed with Peter for two years, and she never once had sexual pleasure. She was in physical pain frequently, but Jennifer felt like she couldn't say no. The price of rejection was too high. She couldn't tell anyone, because she thought that none of her friends were having sex and she didn't want to look like a slut. She also felt Peter betrayed her by being hypocritical to their religious teachings. Most importantly, she betrayed her own values toward sex, her church's values, her parent's values, and her physical body by allowing herself to experience so much sexual pain for so long.

Now, Jennifer is 28. She and her husband have been married 3 ½ years. They had great sex for one to two years when they were

**dating and engaged. Gradually, over the past two years, their sex life has faded to maybe once a month. She loves him, and he loves her. They are both physically attracted to each other. They don't fight much, and if they do, they get over it quickly, except when it comes to sex. There are no deep resentments. She likes sex when she gets into it, but she just avoids sex all the time.**

**Lately, her husband seems to want sex "ALL the time." He is the only one to start sex. She is never interested in making the first move for sex, because she has no interest, and he feels insecure because he doesn't feel she wants him sexually anymore. Now, they hardly ever kiss or hug.**

Jennifer came in for therapy to overcome her negative feelings toward sex and to improve her sex life in her marriage. One of the problems that Jennifer had to overcome was her memory of early bad experiences with sex, partly because she had painful sex for TWO years. She was sexually inexperienced, and she did not want to speak up to Peter when she was having painful sex. Consequently, Peter did not know that what he was doing sexually was actually hurting her, or perhaps he simply didn't pay attention to what was going on with her physically. Since physical pain with first sexual experiences is so common, Chapter 9 will discuss in detail how to avoid painful sex, but besides the physical pain, one of Jennifer's big problems was that she, too, carried a huge amount of guilt for having sex because of her religious beliefs. Even as an adult, she sort of felt like sex was bad, or at least certain kinds of sex, such as oral sex. On top of that, after being betrayed by Peter, she really didn't trust men because of his sexual coercion and his religious hypocrisy.

37

Religious guilt is a very serious concern for many people, so it's important to talk about it at length. Having sexual intercourse before marriage is called fornication, in religious terms, and is believed to be a sin in many religions. But we are wired for sex in our bodies; we are in fact wired to be sexual human beings from birth. We have sexual feelings, but many people are taught not to act on these feelings. Some people are taught that sex is something that God has given us for procreation (to create children), that there can be pleasure from this experience, yet that pleasure is not to be shared until we are married. We discover sexual excitement by seeing, touching, and feeling, ourselves and others, yet we are told by those who are concerned for our well being that sexual activity will be harmful to us. The bottom line is that all of the sexual variations—sex with your self, sex with a married partner, sex with a significant other, or different kinds of sexual interactions—will require a choice each of you will need to make, and some of you will make that decision based on your religious teachings.

> Sex is an act of pleasure, sometimes procreation, and not an obligation!

In some ways, some of the religious teachings, such as the belief that one must be sexually abstinent until marriage, make life and sexuality easier. Life can be less complicated without the problems and possible consequences of sexual interactions, especially if you are a teenager and single. In short, some religious teachings are simply practical advice to help us avoid making decisions that will harm us. Certainly, some of the negative consequences of first sexual experiences, such as getting emotionally hurt by a partner, having complications with relationships, STDs, physical pain, or an unwanted pregnancy, can be avoided simply by staying sexually abstinent, meaning you do not have sexual intercourse at all. Also, there is a definite specialness and beauty in being married to, and sharing a life with, someone who has been and will always be your only sexual partner. This makes a marriage of two individuals very special from an emotional and sexual standpoint. However, you should know that, even without that feeling of specialness that comes from being the "only" sexual partners to each other, within any relationship there is still the capacity to create deep love—emotionally, sexually, and intimately—between two people.

Some religions are very conservative or are called "fundamentalist religions." You may be a part of this type of church or know others who attend these types of churches. For example, someone who attends a fundamentalist church might say, "You will burn in hell if you have sex before you get married." Very conservative or fundamentalist beliefs are based on control, using guilt, shame, and the belief in a punishing God to get people to follow the church's rules and beliefs. This type of religious training can make people feel badly for having sexual feelings, yet some people believe these teachings are God's law and the absolute truth. The sad part is that absolutely everyone has sexual feelings and thus many people end up feeling badly about sex and about themselves. For many teens, this situation makes normal sexual feelings feel frightening. For some teens, it makes them feel like they're choosing between God and sex. While many teens may successfully put down their urges without feeling guilty, others may fail and live with the guilt for the rest of their lives. Frequently in such cases, teens feel they are on their own and must find out the truth about love and sex without God. Remember: God invented sex. Search for your truth with God.

Ideally, it seems wonderful to wait for marriage to become sexually active, but realistically, the truth is that less than one half of girls wait until they are out of high school to have sex. What is important is that, if you have reservations about having sex for religious or spiritual reasons, you need to closely examine these beliefs and act upon them according to what you sense is in your best interest, what is best for you at this point in your life. If you do not feel that you have had your questions answered about what is right for you in the eyes of God, then you need to wait to have sex until it is right for you in order to avoid the resultant guilt. If you are not reasonably sure how you feel about either subject, sex or your religious beliefs, then

Why Don't Girls Want to Have Sex?

you may feel guilty or otherwise bad, and this will make having sex a negative experience for you.

## Parents' Teachings or Parents' Disappointment— Caroline's Story

Caroline's parents had seven children, and she was the seventh child. She knew she was an unwanted pregnancy, an "accident." Her mother had made a joke that she hated hospitals because every time she went to one, they sent her home with a baby! Caroline's mom had her first child at 18, when her dad was 19. Caroline's sex education consisted of one line: "Abstinence is the only way not to get pregnant." Caroline was also told that if she ever got pregnant she would be kicked out of the house and be responsible for taking care of the baby on her own. Caroline looked around at her big family and knew she was not the only "accident." Despite Caroline's minimal sex education from her parents, she stayed away from sex until she was out of high school, despite many opportunities for sexual relationships. Caroline simply did not want to risk pregnancy. She also did not want to disappoint her parents by getting pregnant at an early age, as her mother had, since she watched her mom and dad struggle with raising so many children from the time they were only teenagers.

40

Parents teach you because they love you and want you to be happy and healthy. When parents take the time and energy to teach you about love, sex, relationships, and intimacy, it is because they care about you and want you to avoid getting hurt from relationships and sex. Unfortunately, many parents are also too afraid or embarrassed about sex and relationships themselves to provide complete information to you.

Sometimes the reason parents don't talk to kids about sex is that they don't want to give kids permission to have sex, simply by talking about it. Some parents think that if they talk to you about sex or help you get birth control, then they are telling you it's OK to have sex, when in fact, they want you to wait until you are older or married. Sometimes, as a teenager, *you* too are embarrassed to talk to your parents about these subjects, or you just can't talk to them about anything, period. Plus, most girls are afraid that if they talk to their parents about being sexually active, they'll be banned from seeing their boyfriend again, or even going out. As well intended as parents may be, few parents have the kind of truly open communication with their children that would let them to talk to their teenagers about sexual relationships.

It is important for you to realize that your parents are already communicating to you about relationships and sex, and they have been for many years. This is true whether they are talking to you directly about the subject or not. Every single person reading this book knows their parents well enough to know the extent to which they can talk to their parents about boyfriends, relationships, and sexuality. Most of you know how your parents react to your friends, with whom you are talking on the phone or chatting online, or even if you wanted to see a doctor for birth control.

In fact, parents give you messages about sex from the day you are born. These messages can range from how affectionate your parents are with each other, or with their boyfriends or girlfriends (or lack of them), to their affection with you (are they "touchy-feely" or not?), to what they tell you or don't tell you about dating, talking, and premarital sex. Most teens hear these messages LOUD AND CLEAR and know what the message is without any guessing. More often than not, like values about many other things in life, these values may clash or conflict with your own mind, body and feelings. Perhaps the message is to stay a virgin until you are married. Or to not have a boyfriend until you are 18. Or wait to have sex until you are . . . (fill in the blank).

Caroline's one-and-only message about sex was loud and clear:

"Abstinence is the only sure way not to get pregnant," which was very similar to what my father, who had 10 children, told me. Looking around at *her* six brothers and sisters, Caroline thought her parents might have a good point, and she listened. She decided sex wasn't for her, and this was her only idea about sex for a long time. However, sometimes messages about dating, relationships, and sex come *after* you have already had sexual encounters, and then you tend to feel badly about yourself because it is too late to follow your parents' values.

## Parents and Sex

- **DO** listen closely to your parent's messages and values about sex, if for no other reason than they *do* have your best interests at heart in guiding you in life.
- **DO** know that, frequently, even if you have problems with your parents, and even if you don't agree with a thing they say now, that you will probably understand them and might even agree with their values by the time you are 25. Sometimes, this means that if you rebel against their values you may regret it later.
- **DON'T** hate yourself because you make your own decisions about relationships.
- **DO** know that sometimes your parents will not understand the drives of your heart, your soul, and your mind, and that you have to believe in yourself, balancing your decisions between their guidance and your own knowledge of yourself.
- **DON'T** hate your parents because they don't seem to understand you when it comes to relationships and sex. They may very well understand you or not, but they may still disagree with your behavior, and out of love, they may be trying to help you avoid making a mistake.

## It's Not Enjoyable—Tamika's Story

**Tamika was in 10th grade. She was on the starting team for the Women's Basketball team and very popular with the male basketball players. The girls' team would often help out the guys' team by keeping statistics, setting up the chairs and the benches, and doing announcements for the games. After the games, Tamika usually got a ride home from one of the guys because her mom worked late at night. One of the guys regularly gave her a ride home. Before they went home they would usually go through McDonald's and get something to eat and he would pay for her meal. Tamika kind of felt like she owed this guy something because he was so nice to her, and 'took care of her.' He was attracted to her and after a few rides, he asked her to give him oral sex. She kind of felt flattered that this hot, popular guy, liked her, so at the very beginning she agreed to go along with it. There wasn't much else to the relationship: no kissing, touching, caressing, or talking to each other outside of these situations. Tamika went along with it on several occasions, but she did not like it at all. In particular, she did not like him pushing her head up and down on his penis for oral sex. Tamika was distressed and sought out counseling to talk about it.**

43

Tamika felt she owed this guy something. Although it took a few sessions of counseling, she realized that she did not owe this guy anything, especially sexual favors, for a ride home and a hamburger and coke at McDonald's.

Tamika was pretty disgusted with oral sex and felt used by this guy. Most importantly, she wasn't getting *anything* out of it for herself: she really didn't like this guy that much and she was allowing him to use her. He wasn't kissing or touching her or talking to her, which is what she really liked in relationships. Tamika also didn't realize that giving oral sex was unsafe sex and that she could get a sexually transmitted disease from this behavior. Tamika quickly learned to be more assertive and told the guy she did not want to do it anymore. Sadly, after she turned him down for sex, he wouldn't give her a ride home anymore. This made Tamika feel that she made the right choice, because he was only using her, and she found other rides home.

If you are not having fun with anything you are doing, there is a problem. If you continue to do it and it is not enjoyable, you will be making a bigger problem for yourself now and for yourself in the future. If you are not enjoying it, it's called "bad sex." Too many girls aren't getting anything out of sex, which is a horrible way to lose your virginity and a very good reason for not having sex, even if you're not a virgin.

Why would you want to do something you don't want to do? It's a bad sign if you simply don't like the guy or you're not attracted to him, or if you don't get pleasure from hugging and kissing or sexual contact. Figure out what is happening and/or STOP. Continuing can be very damaging, both physically and emotionally. This includes any kind of physical interaction, even "just giving head," or oral sex. While there are many reasons that girls agree to these things when they do not want to do them, as described in the last chapter, like trying to stay with a guy or to please him, use great caution to treat *yourself* with decency and kindness and to *ensure your enjoyment* in relationships.

## Fear of Pregnancy

As you will read in this book, many girls have unwanted pregnancies, like Suzanna and Georgia. Georgia got pregnant the first time she had sex. Pregnancy, the fear of it, and the reality of the risk, IS REAL. Ninety percent (90%) of teens who are sexually active and do not use birth control will get pregnant within a year of their first sexual experience. YIKES! The risk of an unwanted pregnancy is absolutely a real risk for both young women and young men.

Nearly one in ten teenagers becomes pregnant
before 18.

For these reasons, many girls don't want to have sex or at least
sexual intercourse. No matter how "liberated" a guy might be, *the actual pregnancy happens to girls, and almost always the responsibility either for ending the pregnancy, planning for adoption, or raising a child becomes the sole responsibility of girls.* For teenage girls, only one in nine teen guys who fathers a child is there for her by the end of the pregnancy, in the delivery room. Let's face it, even if you are fairly certain that your boyfriend is Mr. Right, it is very uncommon that he will be Mr. Right There when it comes to pregnancy and birth.

45

Very often guys and young men will just assume that, if you get pregnant, you'll get an abortion, because they do not want to have a baby. If he wants you to have an abortion and you don't agree, you will probably be rejected by him. Most guys will say that if you don't have an abortion, they will not stand by you. Unfortunately, in most cases according to statistics, that assertion is true.

If you get pregnant, you can expect that you will be on your own. You may be lucky to have loving, supportive parents, a great friend, a wonderful sister, or a supportive boyfriend, but the vast majority of girls are on their own, financially and emotionally. Legally, young men are responsible for the financial care of their children through child support, whether they want the child or not, whether they visit the child or not, whether the father is 18 or not. Most states have become better at enforcing child support laws so that fathers really do have to support their children rather than ignoring a court's order to do so. Even if a guy says, "I will never pay child support," it is amazing what a night in jail will do to change a father's mind. If you do decide to have a child, there are more resources and support available for you than ever before in history, but the bottom line is that, if you get pregnant, you will be responsible for caring for this child 24 hours a day, seven days a week, for the next 18 years, unless you are lucky enough to arrange help *sometimes*. This is a hard road, for the best of mothers, so choose wisely.

~~~~~~~~~~

> Always use birth control, or don't have sexual intercourse! Be aware that all birth control methods have some rate of failure.

~~~~~~~~~~

## Timing—Tammy's Story

**Tammy was one of my good friends in high school. She had sex for the first time on the night of her high school graduation with a boyfriend she had loved for over a year. It was just important to her to wait until she finished high school to be sexually active. She felt that, if she had sex in high school, it was too soon for her and she would see herself as a slut. She didn't wait very long after her own "set" time that she felt it was OK to have sex for the first time, actually just a few hours. After the ceremony, when she was 18, she lost her virginity on graduation night, and Tammy was very happy with her decision. Timing was very important for her and, fortunately, her boyfriend respected that choice.**

Timing is sometimes an important factor in a girl's decision not to have sex. When to lose your virginity is a personal decision, and just because the biological clock of your partner says that he wants to have sex or something bad will happen, this does not mean in any way that you should put yourself on their timetable. Your needs and timing for sex are something that you must listen to in a very quiet and reflective manner. Just because your partner wants to have sex now (and later will not do), this should not overrule your sense of the proper timing. Listen to yourself to determine when you feel you are ready or not ready. If your partner really cares about you and wants you to feel good about the experience, then he or she will understand that timing for both of you must be the same or something important will be lost.

Guys do not always understand how girls feel or think about the timing issue. They may think that you are playing a game and just trying to control sex, but in reality you are just trying to be yourself. In truth, you are being controlling: IN CONTROL OF WHAT IS RIGHT FOR YOU! Be true to yourself.

## Awkward or Shy—Carla's Story

Carla was 16 and had her first real boyfriend, "Randy." She had talked to guys online and at school and was "going with guys" in middle school, but she never went past kissing and hugging. Carla was not allowed to start dating until she was 16, when she started going out with Randy. For the first couple of months, they mostly went over to each other's houses, listened to some music, sat outside, watched movies, met each other between classes when they could in high school, and talked on the phone. They had kissed and hugged, and because both of them were attracted to each other, they liked it.

One night they went to a party together at the house of one of Randy's friends, and the parents weren't home. Everyone was drinking a little beer, but no one was being too loud or out of control. Randy and Carla went for a walk together on the property and found a quiet, private place to sit down and talk behind some bushes. Randy started making the moves on Carla and touched her breasts, and then he started to put his hand down her pants. Carla didn't say anything to Randy, but she began to get very nervous. It was Carla's period and she was very embarrassed and too afraid to tell Randy. Suddenly, she got up and ran back to the party. Randy was shocked and ran after her. All Carla could say was that she wanted to go home. Randy took her home immediately, and he apologized to Carla for whatever he did wrong. He thought maybe he went too far, too fast, but Carla didn't even say anything to him because she felt too awkward to tell him about her period. Carla broke up with Randy after this, even though she really liked him, because she just felt too weird at the prospect of talking to him about personal things. Randy never really knew what happened.

**Sex is private.** Yeah, sure, everyone at school and work and on TV talks about sex EVERY DAY. But *your* sexuality is private. Your feelings, your emotions, your crushes, and your thoughts: they are all private. Some people are too private to share this very private part of themselves. Carla had never talked to anyone about anything regarding sex, not even puberty, development, or her periods. Her parents never talked about sex, she didn't have a sister or cousin, or even any close friends. While she had read and heard about things online, her parents had parental controls on the Internet and all her sex ed came from a movie she saw at school in the fifth grade. Carla was simply not comfortable talking about anything of a sexual nature, even something as natural as having a period. Her mom had bought her sanitary pads for her period when she was younger, but they just showed up in the bathroom: there were no discussions or questions asked.

While Carla had spent some time talking to Randy and doing things with him, they never talked about anything private having to do with sex: like periods, or even making out or how far they felt comfortable in going with their sexual explorations. *You need to learn to feel comfortable talking to your boyfriend or girlfriend.* Make friends with them. Go to a coffee shop. Watch a movie. Show up at the same party. Talk. Be friends. Break into a relationship slowly. Sit and have lunch together. Ease into talking about personal subjects. Your comfort level may depend on your previous experience with family relationships and friendships, and if these things were not discussed among your family members then the chances are quite good that you will not feel comfortable discussing them with anyone else either. So, if you are not comfortable with personal and sexual topics, challenge yourself to ease into them a little at a time and practice doing so. In order to have positive first sexual experiences, it is very important to be able to talk about, overcome your shyness, and share what is going on with your feelings.

> Whether you are a teenager or an adult, sex is not the best, and certainly not the most lasting, way to start a relationship: Be friends first!

People who have sex first, then find out later what kind of person their lover is, often regret it and feel embarrassed. Some people who are shy decide to have sex with people without having a relationship because they are too shy to talk. They might think that sex will break the ice or will make the other person like them. While this may work until sex is over, that is when the real awkwardness begins. The participants in very few youthful relationships can continue having sex all the time, especially if you are both living with your parents. So take the opportunity to back up. Learn to talk to people. Address your shyness. If you have a serious problem with sharing your feelings, see a therapist and/or see a psychiatrist. Sometimes shyness has a biological basis and you may need medical help. Group therapy or even joining interactive groups, such as volunteer organizations or sports, can be very helpful as well.

If you feel, in general, too awkward and shy about social situations, then for your own sake, slow down regarding sex. Learn to kiss first, then touch, then *really* touch more, while developing a relationship in which you can talk about having sexual interactions together, and do this until you feel COMFORTABLE. Also, read about sex, talk to your friends, and even talk to your family about it (maybe a friendly aunt or cousin, if you can't talk to your mom or dad or guardians). But please, please, do not go forward with sex with a terrible feeling of embarrassment or

**Why Don't Girls Want to Have Sex?**

awkwardness. It will probably only make you feel worse, sometimes for a long time. This danger alone is a good reason to delay having sex.

## Rumors—Brenna's Story

Brenna was 11 years old. She had a lot of friends in her neighborhood and often rode her bike around, talking to people, socializing and just playing. Some of the guys in the neighborhood built a fort in a small wooded area. It was a really cool fort with two stories that was made out of wood scraps from new houses being built in the area. Brenna would often ride her bike over to the fort and meet with her friends, including boys, even though her parents told her not to go there. Some of the kids had starting smoking in the privacy of the fort, so it was becoming a popular hang out.

One day, Brenna was there with two guys, "Mikel" and "Greg," who were around 14 or 15. The two of them were just sitting in the second story of the fort hanging out. Brenna was sitting between the two of them when they started making some moves on her. They kissed her, and she liked it. Both of them were popular guys and she liked the attention. Then, without asking, and moving quickly at the same time, Mikel put his hand in her button down top and Greg put his hand down her pants, quickly putting his finger inside her vagina. Brenna became very upset and told them to stop, pushing them away from her. They stopped. Still shaking, Brenna thought that was the end of that, ran out of the fort and rode her bike home, but she didn't tell anyone about the experience. She certainly didn't want to tell her parents she was hanging out where she wasn't supposed to be.

A couple of weeks later, Brenna found out that there was a rumor going around that she "went all the way" with two guys at one time in the fort. Brenna was outraged, first because it wasn't true, and second because she felt so embarrassed that everyone was talking about her like she had sex when she was only 11 and going into the 6th grade! Over time, the rumors and taunting from other kids only got even nastier. Mikel was black, and people started calling Brenna, who was white, "a nigger lover," and teasing her with statements like, "Once you go black, you'll never go back, right Brenna?"

To make it worse, Brenna's mother somehow found out about this rumor and asked her about it. Brenna totally lied to her mom and told her it never happened, because she didn't want to get in trouble for being at the fort. Yet, even Brenna's best friend questioned her about what happened and thought that maybe she had done something sexual. It was a terrible summer for Brenna, and she felt like she had been betrayed by these guys who were spreading the rumors, which kept coming up for years.

Brenna came in for therapy in her early 30's. She didn't trust men. This had been her first sexual experience, and it had a negative effect on her opinion about sex from an early age. She did not feel she experienced physical trauma, but she certainly felt emotional trauma that made her not trust men or sex. She was really hurt over the racist comments, too. Brenna didn't have any prejudice about Mikel or black guys, and she was shocked with the racist statements from other white kids. Brenna didn't even realize until she came in for therapy that what she experienced was sexual molestation: she had never consented to the two boys' sexual touching. Yet, for Brenna, the worst part was the rumors that were spread about her and that she had to hear repeated for years afterwards. Even a few years later, people questioned her about liking black guys, and she resented the prejudice over an inter-racial relationship that she didn't even experience.

One of the worst things that girls face, whether they've had sex or not, is the rumor that they have had sex: having people talk bad about your personal business all over school or town.

Why Don't Girls Want to Have Sex?

Big mouths can ruin your reputation, and much of the time the rumors are simply lies. Rumors hurt. Racism hurts. Plus, some guys will only ask you out because they think you put out, and not because they like YOU. Later in this book, we will talk about how you might tell if you can trust someone to keep your private life private.

## Limited Knowledge of Your Own Body and Guys Bodies— Amy's Story

Amy was my grandmother. Her first sexual experiences are prime, although long ago, examples of someone having a very limited knowledge of her body and sex from an early age. Amy's mother had died when she was 11, and her father died when she was 15. She was raised by her uncle and grew up mostly in boarding schools. She knew nothing about physical development or sex. When she started developing breasts earlier than any of her friends in boarding school (and she became quite well endowed), she wrapped her chest in an "Ace" bandage like those used for binding sprained ankles, because she thought she was deformed. When she started having her period at 12, she thought she had cancer and was going to die.

Once, when she was dating in college, a guy offered to teach her how to swim. When he put his arms around her from behind to show her a swimming stroke, she ran away because she was afraid she might get pregnant. She never did learn how to swim. My grandmother got married after her third year of college. While she was in college, she took two years of biology in the 1920's, at Pembroke, an Ivy League school with a good reputation, thinking she would learn the basics of human anatomy and body functions. However, she never learned where babies came from or how they got out of a woman's body until she was actually in the *delivery room* having her first child. Needless to say, it was quite a shock for her. She had many uncomfortable and awkward feelings and experiences, all because she lacked the simplest sex education.

Having a limited knowledge of your body and sexuality, as well as a man's sexuality, can make sex frightening. A lack of knowledge is one reason girls don't want to have sex: they're scared. Most schools provide basic information on health education to help teens understand sexual functioning. Unfortunately, most of the education programs do not provide education on some very important details of sex, such as contraception or ejaculation with oral sex and the potential for the transmission of disease.

In fact, one of my clients did not know what "ejaculate" or "come" really meant. If you don't know either, read Chapter 7 on "Real Sex Education: The Sexual Dictionary." This girl was quite shocked and disgusted when she gave her boyfriend oral sex for the first time and he ejaculated his semen into her mouth. Unprepared, she became very turned off to the idea of oral sex for many years after that. If you do not understand basic stuff about your body and sex, about your partner's body and sex, there is a much higher likelihood that you will have a negative or even traumatic sexual experience. Take the time to know about your body. Also talk to your partner about sex—before, during, and after you have been together—so you will know exactly what is going on.

## Too Nervous

Fear: pay attention to it! Each of us has an internal alarm clock that is there to help us, and it breaks out in a loud noise when we are nervous or afraid. The alarm comes with many different types of signals: a rapid heartbeat, a lump in the throat, a tightness in the chest, a sickness in the stomach, a bad dream, a sudden sweat, and more, depending on the person. Each one of us knows our personal alarm system. If you feel a very big scare about having sex for the first, second, or 50th time; and remember that we are talking about feeling afraid when you are merely thinking about having sex—DON'T DO IT. Closely examine your feelings and thoughts (and even dreams) about sex at this time in your life or with this person who is in your life.

Certainly, if you are with a new partner, you're a virgin, or you're experimenting with sex in a new way, there will be some mild anxiousness and apprehension. In such cases it is probably enough to go slowly until your sense of nervousness is calmed down. But if your internal alarm system goes off and won't shut down, no matter how safe the person or the environment seems: SAY NO . . . and if you need to, GO. In other words, you need to trust that you may understand the situation in which you find yourself even if that understanding is not conscious, even if you can't associate your feelings of alarm with a specific reason.

54

## Fear of Being Naked In Front of Someone Else

A lot of girls feel insecure with being naked in front of someone. Heck, a lot of girls don't feel comfortable being naked in front of a mirror with only themselves in the room! With all the magazines filled with pictures of beautiful, unnaturally thin women blazing half-naked in front of our eyes every day, it is hard to feel confident about our bodies. It is hard to remember that many of these women have been anatomically altered with plastic surgery or that their image has been digitally enhanced by a computer program to make them look that way. Even when you are absolutely beautiful and perfect (whatever that is!), most girls don't know that they look GREAT or even think that they look just OK!

I was a diver on the swim team in high school. I worked out in 12 practices a WEEK! I broke the school record for diving and won at least half of my competitions by my senior year: needless to say, I was in great shape. But I was always worried that I was too fat. At a size nine, I felt HUGE compared to the size 3, 5, and 7 girls. I felt totally inadequate. I look back on my teenage pictures, and honestly, I was in great shape and in fact I was even pretty. But I didn't know it. I was constantly comparing myself to the skinny blonde size

5 girls and feeling overweight. I think about my insecurities at 14, 16 and older, and I just want to cry. It was so sad that these other body images that dominate our culture made me feel that way. In fact, this is really a pitiful reflection of the American culture. Many other countries do NOT have the body image problems that face American girls.

So, if you're like many American girls, it is quite common to feel inadequate about your body . . . even when you are beautiful and perfect. For many girls and women, a poor body image makes it very difficult to feel comfortable about sexuality or sensuality. Read Chapter Six on body image and sexuality for more information. Entire books have been written about this problem, but the bottom line is that you have to feel comfortable with your inner and outer self, your body and your nudity but also how you think and feel, to be comfortable with sex. In the meantime: learn to love your body and take good care of yourself with exercise, nutrition, and good sleep.

## Haven't Found the Right Partner Yet

Yes, research has found that some girls choose not to have sex because they have not found the right partner yet. Some girls are waiting to find the right person before they decide to have a sexual relationship. Waiting for the right person to find the right time for sex for the first time is the #3 reason girls delay sex for the first time. Religious or moral reasons and fear of pregnancy are #1 and #2 (National Center for Health Statistics, 2005.) Waiting for the right person and the right time, saving your virginity for someone special is a very, very good reason to delay sex. Girls who wait until they are over the age of 16, and girls who choose to be abstinent until the right partner is in their life are less likely to regret losing their virginity. So wait, and you won't regret it!

## Fear of STDs

Fear of STDs is the #4 reason some girls delay sex. Chapter 8 discusses STDs, which affect 25% of teenage girls by the time they are 18. Strangely, I have never heard a story from a teenager about delaying sex because of her fear of STDs. Yes, some girls are afraid of AIDS, probably because it is so strongly stressed in the media and even in sex education classes as young as 5th grade, or from personal experience with someone with HIV or AIDS. Yet, I have never, ever heard from a girl that she is afraid of getting an STD to such a degree that she chooses to delay sex. Much more frequently, it seems that most teenagers believe that "it won't happen to them."

Magical thinking takes over when some girls think about sex, believing that HIV and herpes and whatever else those other things are called, "happen to other girls." A myth surrounds sex that STDs happen to "bad girls," or "slutty girls," or to the real "ho" girls. Nothing could be farther than the truth. While it is true that the more sexual partners one has, the more likely one is to be exposed to sexually transmitted infections (also called STI's), all girls who have sex are eligible to get an STD. Even one sexual experience can result in an STD, if your partner has an STD, since when you have sex with someone it is physically like you are having sex with every previous sexual partner they have had! That is why it is very important to protect yourself from STDs each and every time you have sexual contact, which is discussed in detail in Chapter 8.

## WHAT TO DO WHEN YOU'RE NOT READY FOR SEX

**If you don't want to have sexual intercourse, you have a few REAL options:**

1. You can have relationships that do not involve sex at all. Use your sexual voice to speak up about what you want and don't want.

2. You don't have to go out with guys. You can have fun with girlfriends or guy friends, being creative in being joyful!

3. You can have an intimate, loving, sexual relationship with someone without having sexual intercourse, hence, by definition, staying "a virgin" longer. You can share affection by kissing, hugging and touching. You can have all sorts of creative sex with anyone you want to, without having sexual intercourse. "Outercourse" (sexual touch without anal or vaginal intercourse) sex can be GREAT!

4. You can have sex with someone you love: Just you. This is called masturbation, which carries some negative connotations in this culture sometimes, but it is perfectly natural and will help you explore your own notions of sexuality without the inherent physical, emotional, and psychological dangers that accompany sex with a partner. This will be discussed later in Chapter 7.

57

# *three*

# SAME-SEX SEXUAL EXPERIENCES

Having feelings for someone of the same sex can be even more confusing than relationships between girls and guys. At some point in their lifetimes, many people have feelings for, attractions to, or experiences with someone of the same sex. This chapter helps you to understand and deal with some of the experiences girls have with same sex relationships. Homosexuality is a label that describes sexual attraction for, sexual desire to, or sexual behaviors with a person of one's own sex, but most people use the words "gay" or "queer" to describe same sex sexual relationships, so that is what is used in this book. "Lesbian" is a word for a woman who is gay. Throughout this book, sexual partners are often referred to as "guys" or "boyfriends," but please know that *Virgin Sex* refers to a sexual partner of any gender, including someone of the same sex or a transgendered person (someone who feels like they were born with the wrong sexual parts).

## Debbie and Alice's Story

**Debbie and Alice went to a small, private Presbyterian college in**

Austin, Texas in 1977. They became friends their freshman year of college. Debbie had dated guys, but she had always had crushes on girls ever since she could remember, from as early as the 1st grade. However, she had never had any sexual experiences with girls, not even kissing. In 1977, being gay was even more 'taboo,' or against the rules of society, than it is today. Debbie really didn't know how to talk to a girl about having a crush on her, or even how to know if she herself was gay or not, let alone if the other girl was gay. It was very confusing and frustrating. Consequently, Debbie had a crush on Alice a long time before she ever acted on her feelings. It is very hard to have feelings toward someone of the same sex, because you don't necessarily know if they are gay, and you are very afraid that if you tell them you are gay you will be rejected for that simple reason alone. As with other relationships, you also are afraid of simply not being liked. Then, if they're not gay, and they're homophobic [afraid of homosexuality], you might lose the friendship you may have shared with this person, too. So, like many people who have feelings toward someone of the same sex, neither Debbie nor Alice said anything to each other for a long time.

At college, Debbie and Alice drank a lot of alcohol and also experimented with marijuana. One night, when they were both very drunk and high, they were goofing around and a friend of theirs threw them both on the bed. They were just lying there, intoxicated, and found themselves in the bed, together and alone. They rolled toward each other and began kissing. Each of the girls responded to the other, because Alice had actually had a crush on Debbie for a long time too but never said anything. Alice had never had a sexual relationship with a woman, either. They ended up making love, and it was a wonderful, exciting thing for both of them. After that night, they fell totally in love with each other and continued their sexual relationship. It was the most fantastic relationship for both of them, because for the first time in their lives they both felt in love and happy.

While both of these young women had dated men, there had

been something missing: love. Alice and Debbie found out that love put the love in lovemaking. It was a new and wonderful relationship. They were so happy, and it was so obvious that they told all their friends they were in love and happy. That is when the sexual experience became very negative, however.

It was a very small school, and just like small towns, everyone talks and everyone seems to know everything about everyone else. Within a few weeks, everybody on campus found out they were gay and rejected them. Now remember, this was 1977, and being gay was even less acceptable than it is today. For Debbie and Alice, even their best friends and acquaintances would have nothing to do with them and wouldn't talk to them or hang out with them anymore. They were ostracized on the whole college campus.

At first, Debbie and Alice didn't care. They were totally in love. They had each other, did everything together, and they were ecstatic in their own world. But then, Alice's roommates told her to move out of their apartment because she was gay. Alice began to feel the isolation of having no friends on campus or even in her own apartment, and she quickly became afraid that she wouldn't have a place to live. Reluctantly, Alice decided to break off her relationship with Debbie.

Debbie was completely crushed. She was isolated, because no one would talk to her or even hang out with her. She felt confused and sad about being gay, which reflected her own sexual identity and therefore who she was as a person. She decided she didn't want to live anymore. Devastated, Debbie tried to kill herself by taking an overdose of pills.

Fortunately, Debbie survived the suicide attempt. She spent some time in a psychiatric hospital, where she nevertheless continued to feel depressed and lonely. Ultimately, she did return to campus and got counseling from the minister at the school. The female pastor was very supportive and helpful. Debbie also talked to the minister about having been date raped during her freshman year.

When Debbie was a freshman, she had been dating a guy and

went to his place for a party. She became very drunk during the party, so she went to her boyfriend's room to lie down. His roommate came into the room and raped her. Debbie went to the Student Union at the campus and reported the rape. This was (and still is) a very hard thing to do, to tell someone you have been raped, especially if it is at a small college and everyone finds out about it. It was also hard to do because she had been drunk, which made her feel somewhat responsible for the rape. She was in no way responsible in reality of course, but she felt that she had put herself in a bad position by being drunk and being in the roommate's bedroom. Although she did have the courage to report the rape, the school did nothing to act on the rape charges. The school officials told her there was nothing they could do, because she had been very drunk, she was in the guy's bedroom, and they couldn't prove anything. Sadly, the school swept the whole situation under the rug, and they did what happened to all too many young women in the 1970s who had been raped: They blamed the victim! The school's behavior was disgusting, but sadly, this certainly was not an unusual reaction.

After several weeks, Debbie and Alice got back together. Their love for each other meant that they just couldn't be kept apart. They decided to live together in Debbie's dorm room. When the college found out, the campus officials then kicked them off campus because they were gay and living together.

In 1977, in Austin, Texas, you could live on campus and be a rapist, but you couldn't live there if you were in love and gay!

Debbie and Alice both had a very difficult time in college in their struggle with homosexuality. As you can see, Debbie suffered through drug addiction, suicide, rejection from her friends, and a lack of support from her college. Despite their problems, Debbie and

Alice stayed together for a few years. They found other gay people in the community, moved in with one of them, and found another gay couple with whom to be friends. This made life a lot easier and they were a lot happier. Although they later broke up, they grew up a lot and helped each other struggle with being gay and being generally unaccepted by people at the college, in their workplaces, and by their families.

The good news is that both Debbie and Alice are now openly gay and their families have accepted them. Both of them are very successful. Debbie is a counselor, who specializes in the treatment of drug addiction. Alice is a successful lawyer, who helps many gay people with their legal struggles, problems that include asserting gay parents' rights.

Although it has been many years since Debbie and Alice's struggles with being a gay couple in the 1970s, some things have gotten better in our society for gays and lesbians but some haven't changed. Recently a gay woman, in a large college in South Carolina, was living in a dorm room with her girlfriend. The two of them had to move out because the dorm had turned into an all sorority dormitory. When they looked for a new placement on campus, they were only given the choice to go to an all-black girl's dormitory because they were considered "misfits." They were told there were "no other placements available to *them*." This was in the year 2000!

## Jodie's Story

**Jodie knew she was different ever since she could remember being a person, from around 5 years old. She was always attracted to girls, not to boys. She, of course, kept this a secret, as it was quickly obvious that other girls only talked about boys: how cute they were, whether or not they were looking at you, whether or not they liked you. In middle school, she had several crushes on girlfriends, but mostly she kept them to herself. On a couple of occasions, she told**

girls she liked them. On both of these occasions, however, the girls in question in middle school rejected her and told her they weren't her friends anymore. So she stopped telling people about her crushes. In high school, Jodie had a crush on the school gym teacher. It turned out, as Jodie wrote, "She was the one gym teacher who wasn't gay, LOL." Actually, Jodie felt very isolated, alone, different, and confused. She knew she was gay, but she had no idea how to be gay or to find someone else who was also gay. Her early attempts to share her feelings with girls were dismal failures, and the aftermath was loaded with people talking behind her back and no one telling her they liked her in return.

Jodie's first sexual experience was with a boy. Even though Jodie knew she liked girls and not guys, she decided to go out with a guy because it was what everyone else was doing. After all, Jodie was a cute, petite girl with an athletic figure, not "butch" looking, and guys were attracted to her. As a teenager, at least someone was attracted to her, and she wanted to be liked and given attention! As Jodie describes herself, she was "70% feminine and 30% butch." So, wanting some intimate attention, Jodie went out with a few guys, and her first sexual experience with a guy was when she was 17.

She and "Marty" went out on a date and ended up parking somewhere to make out. During this make out session, "Marty" put his finger in her vagina and "IT HURT—BAD!" The date ended quickly after that, but the event lasted for a long time in Jodie's mind. She knew she didn't like what guys had to offer and didn't want to go any further with that.

Jodie's first sexual experience with a woman, at 18, was not any better, though! This time, Jodie was attracted to the girl and was interested in sexual experimentation. They kissed and touched. Touching led to the same thing as it had with Marty, with "Liz" putting her finger inside her. "IT HURT AGAIN!" This sex thing was not very much fun and didn't feel good to Jodie. It made her feel even more confused about her sexual identity.

Same-Sex Sexual Experiences

Liz and Jodie were very sexually inexperienced and did not know the first thing about having loving sexual touching: tender, arousing, and *slow-going at first*. As a result, Jodie didn't like sex and felt confused about sexual desire, attraction and her sexual identity.

In college and afterwards, Jodie had different and positive sexual experiences, but her early experiences caused her to have a lot of emotional pain about sex, fear about sexual pain, and confusion over her sexual identity. These years of confusion and pain were unnecessary, if only she were more educated about sex, and particularly about being gay.

First of all, Jodie was confused about whether or not she was gay. In the next section, guidance is provided to help girls explore whether or not they are gay or bisexual. Second, Jodie was confused because she had sexual interactions with both a guy and a girl, *neither* of which were pleasurable. This made her uncertain of her sexual identity. Many people are confused about what they like and don't like when it comes to sex, whether they are gay or straight. However, many girls, even when they are attracted to the same sex, don't know what lesbians are supposed to do when they make love. A lot of straight adults wonder what lesbians do when they make love, too.

## SO WHAT IS LESBIAN SEX?

Remember: lesbians are people, and they are women who are sexual. Lesbian sex is about sharing love and sexual pleasure in whatever way two people decide to connect emotionally, physically and spiritually. Lesbians can enjoy romance, companionship, kissing, hugging, touching, caressing, oral sex, vaginal penetration, and anal stimulation. Lesbians enjoy the same type of sexual pleasuring and variation that any other woman would enjoy, except they enjoy it with another woman. Lesbians have likes and dislikes with sex, just like straight girls. Most lesbians like oral sex, some don't, some like vaginal penetration with a finger, some don't. Lesbians do like to have orgasms, just like other women: some have them, some don't. Lesbians like orgasms from having their clitoris touched, some like orgasms from vaginal penetration, with a finger or tongue or sexual toy, but some don't. Lesbians love to love their partners and they love enthusiasm! Mostly, lesbians want to love and be loved, which is the greatest gift on Earth.

## HOW DO I KNOW IF I AM GAY OR BISEXUAL?

Knowing "for sure" if you are gay can be very confusing. Some people "know" they are gay from a very young age, because they have always and almost exclusively had attractions to members of their same sex. For many people, figuring out your sexual orientation is a process of discovery, with much uncertainty along the path. Generally, a person who is gay is attracted to members of the same sex and desires or has sexual experiences with someone of the same sex. Generally, a person who is bisexual is sexually attracted and interested in having sexual relationships with girls and guys. However, many people have occasional attractions or sexual fantasies or sexual experiences with members of the same sex when they do not identify themselves as gay or bisexual. Recent research shows that 11% of teens have a same sex sexual experience, although it is more common with Black and White girls than Hispanic girls (6%). It is estimated that 20–30 percent of women have a same-sex sexual experience in their lives.

Being gay or bisexual is not a black or white situation. An attraction to the same sex may include feeling in love with someone, having fantasies about them, feeling sexual desire for them, or having sexual behavior with them. Attraction works like a scale on a number line:

65

| Heterosexual | | | | | | Homosexual |
|---|---|---|---|---|---|---|
| 1 | 2 | 3 | 4 | 5 | 6 | |

When a person is asked, on a scale from one to six, "Do you see yourself as heterosexual or homosexual, including having love, fantasies, desires, or sexual behaviors?" about 90% of people see themselves as a 2, 3, 4 or 5. The minority of people see themselves as exclusively or only heterosexual or homosexual, in their thoughts, feelings and behaviors. For example, a girl who sees herself as a "2" might only be attracted to guys and fantasize about having sexual experiences with guys, but she may find herself being attracted to looking at women's breasts and getting a little turned on without ever wanting to act on this attraction. A girl who sees herself as a "5" may only be attracted to girls, and identify herself as gay, but she may have had a sexual experience with a guy. Many people have sexual fantasies, sexual desires or attractions to members of the same sex, but they may never act on them or want to act on them with sexual behaviors. Being attracted to or having an occasional fantasy with someone of the same sex does not mean you want to have a sexual experience with them or that you are gay.

Being gay is more than just having a sexual experience with another person of the same sex. It means being connected to another person of the same sex physically, spiritually, and emotionally. When this happens, the experience tells a person who they are and what they are. Many people find that having a romantic, fun, or sexual experience with a person tells them a lot about who they are. If you are confused about feelings toward another girl, especially if you have acted on those feelings sexually, give yourself this little test:

# The Mini After 'Date' Quiz

- How did you feel with this person?
- Was it exciting?
- Was it "all that?"

For gay people who have heterosexual experiences (and for straight people who have gay experiences), the emotional and/or sexual feelings regarding the experience may be one of big disappointment or "flatness," an overall lack of excitement with the experience. Then, when they have a homosexual (or heterosexual) experience, they feel much more turned on, much more excited, much more understanding of why people even WANT to have both romance and sexual experiences. In other words, this particular version of sexual experience "does it for them." There is a feeling of, "This is it! This is what I like! This is who I am."

Whether you are gay or straight, also remember the types of feelings you have, both emotionally and physically, will depend on your attraction to an *individual*. Sometimes people have initial dating and sexual experiences with someone to whom they have a weak attraction. Or maybe there is a strong physical attraction, but the person hasn't been very nice to you or treated you badly in some way. Or maybe you are not very physically attracted to the person, but you just love their personality and you are drawn to that person for that reason alone. The degree of physical attraction and emotional attraction (or repulsion) will have a big effect on how much you like dating, sharing activities, kissing, touching, and having sexual experiences with this particular person.

Sometimes people are attracted to someone simply because of their personality or general spirit, not because of their body or their genital parts. This may only happen once in a lifetime, and people

67

wonder, "Does this mean I'm gay?" If you get into a sexual relationship with the person, literally, it does mean you have had a gay or bisexual experience. But many "gay" people don't feel "gay" as if the experience were utterly different from feeling non-gay: they just happened to fall in love with a person of the same sex. It happens, and it can be confusing when this happens. Some people have the courage to express and enjoy the love they have found in their lives; some people don't. I just say to such a confused client, "If you can love men and women, you can . . . if you can't, you can't." Those people who can love both men and women may identify themselves as bisexual, but some don't. Sometimes they just consider a certain experience an isolated event and don't try to label themselves at all. As stated above, many people have sexual experiences at least once with a member of the gender outside their usual choice, with both men and women.

Sometimes, there is no explanation to when and for whom we feel love or to whom we feel attracted. You can't help who the person happens to be to whom you are attracted: it just happens and the feelings are involuntary. Sometimes it means you are gay, and sometimes it doesn't. Of course, if you are always attracted to people who are bad for you, like people who beat on you, physically or emotionally, or to people who are alcoholics, it is time to see a counselor or therapist and work on this problem, to figure out why you are attracted to people who hurt you rather than to someone who gives you joy. You do not need to see a therapist just because you are attracted to someone of the same sex. Most therapists and researchers agree that therapy can't change your sexual orientation. Yet, therapy might help you deal with your problems with family, friends and society accepting you, or indeed it might help you accept yourself and the attraction you are feeling.

## SPECIAL ADVICE ON BEING GAY AND HAVING SEX FOR THE FIRST TIME

Sex for the first time, if you think or know you are gay, has a lot of things in common with the first sexual experiences of people who are not gay. For one, attraction is important. Being with someone because you are attracted to them makes love and sexual encounters special. Second, every person has their own personal conditions for sexual experiences. As we'll discuss in the next chapter, these conditions may include having a committed and exclusive relationship, being in love, being a certain age, being in a certain environment, or having a deeply trusting partner. Paying attention to your conditions for sex is very important for having positive sexual experiences.

69

Simply being heterosexual, or straight, means you do not have to question convention. The hard thing about being gay is that it means redefining your entire sexuality and your relationship with society. As some of you may have already found out, being gay is not generally accepted at home, in your church, at your school, or even among your friends. In fact, in many parts of the world, being gay results in being rejected by virtually everyone, just because you are attracted to someone of the same sex.

## COMING OUT

Coming out means letting people know you are gay or bisexual. The decision to come out can be, and in fact is, the subject of entire books, and I encourage you to search out these resources. The first consideration in coming out is coming out to yourself. Often people spend years, alone, contemplating their sexuality and being too scared to talk to anyone about it for fear of being rejected. Rejection is a reality in our society when you are gay. For many gay people, rejection, or the fear of it, makes them feel entirely isolated, depressed and even suicidal.

> You need to have someone to talk to about being gay!

Being isolated and feeling you don't belong is no way to go through high school, college, or life. First come out to yourself, at least to the extent that you admit to yourself that you are thinking about or are attracted to members of the same sex.

Next, you need to find someone with whom to talk. Finding someone to talk to will make a huge difference in your life. Some people are lucky enough to have accepting parents and friends. With my sons, and since they were young boys, as a preface to any discussion about sex I've always said, "When you are older, and dating, a girl or a guy . . . " With my daughter, I would say, "When you have a boyfriend or a girlfriend . . . " I wanted my children to feel like it would be OK if they were straight, gay, or bisexual. I really didn't care if they were gay or not, I just wanted them to have the experience of loving and being loved, and I wanted them to be happy.

Many parents, teachers, preachers, and people in society don't feel this way, however. Many people feel homosexuality is a sin. Many people quote the Bible as saying, "Same-sex acts are sinful." However, some gay churches interpret the Bible differently than this or choose to believe that God will love them, no matter whom they love. Of course, this is a big controversy for our society, and the bottom line is that a lot of people reject homosexuality, but not all people do.

You need to find someone to talk to who does not reject you for being gay, someone who will talk to you about it. It can be very hard to find such a confidant, or even to have any idea where to look for such a person. Sometimes parents are open to talking to you about your

70

feelings. You probably already know their feelings about homosexuality. You know if your parents or guardians are "gay friendly" or not.

If your parents or guardians aren't open, you may be able to turn to your friends. You can "test" your parents or friends for their ability to accept or reject you by just talking about someone gay or by discussing a story or movie on homosexuality, such as *The Philadelphia Story*, to see how they react. Even if there is a positive response, however, you should know that you will be taking a risk in sharing a very private part of yourself: your sexuality. You should know that, although they might generally tolerate homosexuality, they might be freaked out if they know *you* are gay. You should also know that a LOT of parents and friends ALREADY know or suspect that you might be gay. In most of these situations, they are afraid to say anything to you in case you aren't gay, because they don't want to hurt your feelings. This means that, sometimes, people are really prepared to talk to you and accept you. Other family members may also be possible candidates for someone to share your feelings with, such as an aunt or uncle, a cousin, or even a grandparent.

If your parents or friends are in no shape to talk to you about your sexuality, you will need to consider coming out to someone else. One option may be a school counselor or teacher. Keep in mind that counselors are required *by law* to maintain the full confidentiality of anything you talk to them about (except for threats to kill one's self or someone else). Teachers do not have to abide by a law of confidentiality, however, and if you absolutely do not know if you can trust them, try a counselor instead. If your school counselor will just not do, you may try your pastor or minister. A minister is also bound by confidentiality and can't tell anyone what you talk about. If you do not attend church, or if you belong to a very conservative church, this may not work, either. You might also ask your parents to take you to a counselor or therapist. You can go to a community mental health center for free, and many medical insurance companies will pay all or a portion of the cost for a private therapist. If the counselor is obviously NOT gay-friendly (which most counselors are trained to be), then find another one. Find one with whom you feel comfortable and to whom you can talk about anything.

If you can't find anyone in your immediate family or a counselor to talk to, try to find a gay or lesbian group in the community. Most community newspapers have weekly listings for gay or lesbian support groups or churches. If there is a community college or university in your area, contact general information at the school and most will have a GLBT (gay, lesbian, bisexual, transgendered) support group. If none of these options work, go to the Internet. There are MANY resources on the Internet for gays and lesbians, including resources specifically for teenagers. The Internet is a great way to discover yourself and to gain free information, but as with any contact with a new person or organization, you obviously need to be careful that the information is accurate and the intentions of the people on the other end of your communication are trustworthy. See Chapter 10 on Do's and Don't of the Internet. There are also gay and lesbian teen chat rooms to connect with other teens, and often, these resources are a great place to start before even trying to talk to another person face to face. However, connecting with someone electronically does not replace having a personal connection with someone in your life who will support you. Please remember that the Internet, or your use of it from your home, may not be completely private: every communication is potentially traceable. If you have a concern that someone may be monitoring your Internet use, you may want to use a public library or another public resource.

*four*

# HOW DO I KNOW IF
# I'M READY FOR SEX?

A s you can see from reading the stories in Chapters 1, 2, and 3, many girls have sexual experiences before they are really ready for sex. This chapter helps you decide if YOU are ready for a sexual relationship or experience. This chapter is designed to help you think about what is right for YOU and to make the best decision about sexual experiences: physically, emotionally and spiritually. The following quiz is a good place to begin thinking about what you need in order to be ready for sex. Each of the items in this quiz will be discussed at length to help you look at the many considerations of having a sexual relationship.

> If you answer no to any of these questions, then you need more time and preparation to really be ready for sex.

## Dr. Darcy's Am I Ready for Sex? Quiz

1. Are My "Conditions" For Sex Met?

2. Is Having Sex Now Who I Am : Not What Someone Else Wants?

3. Do I Know My Body Well Enough To Have Sex?

4. Am I Sure I Am Not Confusing Sex With Love?

5. Can I Handle Possible Rejection And The Emotional Consequences Of Sex?

6. Have My Boyfriend And I Considered What We Would Do If I Got Pregnant?

7. Am I Ready To Use Birth Control And Practice Safer Sex?

8. Am I Comfortable Enough With My Partner To Talk About Sex?

9. Can My Partner And I "Legally" Have Sex?

10. Would I Have Sex If I Weren't Drunk Or High?

## 1. ARE MY "CONDITIONS" FOR SEX MET?

In Chapter 1, the story of "Jon" was about a guy who wanted to have sex because he had a chance at having sexual intercourse with one of the hottest girls in school. Jon was physically attracted to Amber, but he just couldn't physically, sexually "perform." He couldn't get an erection because he didn't feel like he should be "taking" Amber's virginity when he didn't have any emotional feelings for her. Although this may sound really hard for some people to believe because it is about a young man having qualms about sex with a beautiful girl, this is a TRUE story: this guy couldn't "get it up" because he felt like the situation was wrong for him.

VIRGIN SEX *for Girls*

You have to look at your own values, needs, and feelings to determine what your conditions are for sex. Everyone has different ideas of what is important to them when it comes to making love or having sexual experiences with someone.

## What Are My Conditions For Sex?

- Do I need to be in love with him or her?

- Does he or she need to be in love with me?

- Do I need to be "going out" with him or her for a certain length of time?

- Do I only need to be physically attracted to him or her?

- Do I need to be in an "exclusive" relationship (meaning that neither of you have other girlfriends or boyfriends)?

- Do I need to have a trusting relationship?

- Is open, comfortable communication important to me?

- Do my partner or I need to be a certain age?

- Do we need to be of the same race or religion?

- Do we need to be engaged or married?

- Does this have to be the person I plan to spend my life with?

- Do we want to have sex during my period?

- Am I OK with having a "one night stand" (meaning you have sex one time and never plan on seeing each other again or having a relationship)?

Make sure your conditions for having sex are met, or you may be angry with yourself later. Sometimes, if people don't meet their conditions for sex, they feel guilty, dirty, shameful, regretful or even blame their partners and mess up their relationships. Sex is for *you and your partner.*

~~~~~~~~~~~

Make sure your values, needs, feelings and
conditions for sexual experiences are met!

~~~~~~~~~~~

## 2. IS HAVING SEX NOW WHO I AM: NOT WHAT SOMEONE ELSE WANTS?

Remember the stories of Jayne, Melissa, and Kayla from Chapter 1? Jayne had sex to please her boyfriend, Juan, which always meant giving him "blow jobs." Melissa had sex to keep her boyfriend, and after having sex with him, he expected her to "put out" all the time. Neither Jayne nor Melissa really wanted to do what they did. For Jayne, the experience resulted in her crying whenever she had sex, even into her 20s. For Melissa, the experience made her feel used every time she had sex. On the other hand, Kayla felt she wanted to have sex just because she felt like she was ready. She also felt in love with her boyfriend. She felt like she had a good time and had a lot of positive feelings about sex in her life.

You have to ask yourself if *you* are really ready to have sex for *you*. If you don't ask this question of yourself, sex will be a compromise of who you are, and the effects of this compromise can last for many years.

Sometimes, it is the guy who pressures you into sex. Sometimes, however, it is your friends. If a friend puts pressure on you or teases you continually because you are a virgin, then they're not your friend. A friend will respect you for who you are, including who you are sexually. Sometimes friends can make *you* put pressure on yourself to lose your virginity, although if you really look at what you want and who you are, you might find it is you trying to please your friends rather than doing what you want. Just being able to say you are no longer a virgin is not going to make you feel any better about yourself than you did when you were a virgin, especially if you

76

have sex in the wrong situation, for the wrong reasons, and with the wrong person.

~~~~~~~~~~~~~~~~~

You will always remember your first sexual experiences.

~~~~~~~~~~~~~~~~~

You want to be proud when you remember that your first experiences reflected your personal desires, who you are, and your own sense of timing, even IF, in the long run, YOU decide that you made a mistake when you look back at the circumstances. That is, you need to know in the future that you made the best choice you could with the knowledge you had about yourself, sex and your partner at the time. At least you can say, "I did it MY WAY." You want sex to be special for you, not something you did just to "get it over with" or to prove something to your friends. Really, most good friends secretly wouldn't respect you doing something that you didn't feel was right for yourself anyway. Another truth is that many of those same people who are driving you to have sex secretly regret their first sexual experiences, but they're not likely to tell you because they don't want to admit it to anyone, perhaps not even to themselves.

In Chapter 1, both Janice and Anna had sex because their friends were doing it, and they thought they should be, too. For Janice, because she didn't want to have sex, she learned to not like sex and "turned off her sexual switch." She even got married and still didn't like sex. Her husband had an affair because she didn't want sex. This ended their marriage. The long-term consequences of doing it because her friends were doing it were negative for Janice. It took a lot of therapy and examination of her life for Janice to figure out how to "turn the sexual switch" back on.

Anna lived with the lie of telling her friends she was sexually active for more than two years. After a while, she couldn't live a lie, and she decided to have sex with a guy who really did not care about

77

her only so she would no longer be a virgin. Anna felt so badly about her experience that she became an alcoholic. Anna also had a terribly embarrassing and dangerous situation by getting so drunk while she was babysitting that she had to be taken away in an ambulance. Later, she had a bad sexual relationship with her husband. Anna stayed with her husband, however, who was a really nice guy. He was patient and tried to understand her problems from the past, but her feelings about sex did cause many years of pain for her before she got help. The worst part is that Anna never really felt loved *for herself*. It took her a long time to accept that her husband loved her for her and not just for sex, and even longer to love and respect herself.

Ask yourself: Are you having sex just to be popular?

Popularity has to do with a lot of different things, depending on your community, your school, and your friends. Feeling good about yourself, what we call self-esteem, is something that you earn—you don't just get it from having sex. In fact, sex can have the opposite effect and leave you feeling the only thing you are liked or known for is sex. Is that really what you want to be known for? Working on finding your natural talents and gifts and using them is what really makes you feel good about yourself. Self-esteem comes from doing "esteemable acts."

Self-esteem is earned from you being you, and being good at it, not from doing what other people think you should do.

In Chapter 1, we talked about Georgia, who had sex with her boyfriend for the "special occasion" of his going off to war. The sexual relationship resulted in an unexpected pregnancy (and a bad marriage that followed). From time to time, many girls feel pressured by themselves or their partners to have sex just because it is a special occasion, such as celebrating their birthday, winning a basketball championship, or going to the prom. Sometimes, you may really feel that you love your boyfriend, and he may not be pressuring you for sex, but you sort of feel like you "owe it" to him because he's your boyfriend.

## "SPECIAL" GUIDELINES FOR SEX

- If you WANT to have sex with your boyfriend because it is a special occasion, AND you're ready for sex, it can make sex for the first time special.

- If you DON'T WANT to have sex, you don't "OWE" anyone sex.

- If you want to be sexually intimate with your boyfriend, but you are not ready for sexual intercourse, try outercourse: sexual sharing without penis/vagina penetration.

- If you are with someone who thinks sex is an *obligation*, reconsider the relationship, even if you feel you love them, because they're not respecting YOUR needs and may not be LOVING YOU.

Sex is a mutual sharing of physical intimacy, NOT an obligation. Read the stories about the girls in Chapter 1 who were having sex just because they were trying to please their boyfriends and ignored their own feelings, wants, and desires. Having sex because they felt they had an obligation caused them to be messed up about sex for a long time.

Remember: Your sexuality is special and it needs to be special for you, too.

## 3. DO I KNOW MY BODY WELL ENOUGH TO HAVE SEX?

To know whether or not you are ready for sex, you will need to know your body well enough to have sex. Many girls think that guys will know more about a girl's body than she will, and many girls depend upon the guy to get them turned on. But girls need to know what gets them turned on, how to get themselves turned on, and be confident enough to tell a guy what they want or like.

> If you do not know your own body, you are not physically ready for sex!

It is a girl's responsibility to know what she likes and what she doesn't like. It is not a guy's responsibility. If you do not know your own body, what it likes, and how it responds, you will be at risk for giving a guy control over you. You want to be in control of yourself first, then you can share what you like with someone else who is enthusiastic to learn about you. Plus, you might change what you want physically and sexually depending on the day or on your mood. You need to let your partner know what you are in the mood for on any particular day.

At first, you will not know how you will respond to being with a partner in a physical way, because you can't always predict your response. In your first physical experiences with guys, kissing and touching will be new and you really will not know how you feel until you have this experience. Take time with a partner to experience kissing and touching each other in many ways, or with different partners over time, just to see what you like. You will begin to get an idea about what you like. For example, you may find you like French kissing on the mouth and in your ear, even though that may sound gross right now. Or you may like to have your breasts touched but not your nipples pinched. After a period of exploration, you will get to know your own feelings from kissing and touching. Most of the time this exploration will lead to physical feelings of sexual excitement. You need to understand and be comfortable with your feelings of sexual excitement, and you need to learn what feels good to you prior to having sexual intercourse.

It is essential that you know what parts of your body you like to have touched, or not touched, and that you share this information with your partner. Your partner may love you very much, and he may even have some ideas of touching or physically relating which are new and interesting to you. However, no partner is a mind reader, and if you don't know yourself physically and share this personal information with your partner, you are going to miss out on the best parts of physical and sexual interactions: WHAT YOU LIKE.

Girls can also learn what they like with physical feelings and sensations through self-touch. In Chapter 6, we will talk more fully about self-touch. This means a girl can explore her own body and find out what feels good to her. Later, if you want to, you will be able to share your self-knowledge with another person with greater confidence.

Physically, most girls are able to have sexual intercourse after puberty. However, every girl is made differently, and every girl's body is different, including her size and her physical responses to sexual touch. So, it only makes sense that every girl will be physically ready for sex at different times and for different reasons. Every girl's vagina is a different size, and the variation is even more pronounced when girls are young or not fully developed at the end of puberty. As a general rule of thumb, most girls are not fully developed until they are 16. In fact, because girls' vaginas are not fully developed at a cellular level, girls younger than 16 are more likely to get STDs!

Sexual penetration is easier and more pleasurable physically when you are sexually excited or aroused. To be physically ready for sex, first you must be physically aroused. In order to get physically aroused, you need to know what turns you on, or sexually excites you. A lot of girls don't know how to get aroused or know when they are turned on.

Physically, there are some signs of being turned on: your vagina gets lubricated or "wet," sometimes your heart beats faster, sometimes there is a red flush on your chest, sometimes it is just a feeling of being 'horny' or sexually excited. Some girls get turned on from simply kissing, hugging or touching. Other girls may need more direct sexual stimulation of the genitals by the touch of a hand or mouth. Chapter 6 will talk more fully about physical arousal and sexual responses to touch.

A sexual myth: It is not true that a girl's vagina can accommodate any size penis!

Most girls are taught in health or sex ed class that, physically, any man's penis can fit into any girl's vagina. However, the truth is that sometimes a guy's penis is simply too big to fit into a girl's vagina. In fact, while most guys don't know this, many more women complain that a guy is too big than complain that a man is too small. The following is true for *all girls*: when you are a virgin, you will need to physically prepare yourself for intercourse in order to have physical pleasure when you have sex for the first time. At first, sex needs to be a slow process of physically preparing your body for intercourse. This is fully explained in detail in Chapter 9 in the section that discusses how to have sexual intercourse with minimal or no physical pain. The basic idea is that your vagina needs to be slowly introduced to having penetration with touch long before penetration occurs using an erect penis.

## 4. AM I SURE I AM NOT CONFUSING SEX WITH LOVE?

In Chapter 1, the story of Suzanna tells about her seeking love through sexual relationships. Sometimes sexual experiences provide an intimacy that makes someone feel loved . . . at least during the experience. Often, later, as in Suzanna's case, a girl might find out that the guys she was with really just wanted to have sex and they weren't interested in love or having a relationship. Are you really wanting sex? Or are you really wanting to be loved? Wanting to be loved is one of the most common reasons girls have sex when they are not ready. It is easy to confuse love with sex, because sex can make you feel very intimate and close with someone. Sex can be "lovemaking," an act of sharing and expressing your love together, but if someone really loves you, you will feel it, whether you have sex or not. If love is not there before sex, the closeness of sexual feelings will not last and sex won't make someone love you.

> When love is true, you can truly make love. But sex doesn't make love and you can't make love out of sex.

## 5. CAN I HANDLE POSSIBLE REJECTION AND THE EMOTIONAL CONSEQUENCES OF SEX?

You need to consider all of the potential emotional consequences of sex and be ready to deal with them. The biggest one is being emotionally rejected or hurt. The most common ways that girls are emotionally hurt are as follows:

- Being rejected or breaking up with your boyfriend. A lot of guys just want to have sex with girls, and they have no intention of having a relationship.
- Sex can also change a relationship in that girls tend to have more expectations for a deeper emotional commitment to a relationship, especially after things get sexual. Some guys want this deepening of the relationship and some don't even know how to do this. If the two of you want different things, you can get hurt.
- Almost all teenage relationships end. Can you handle taking the reality of loving and losing love?

**How Do I Know If I'm Ready for Sex?**

- Not having privacy with your boyfriend about sex. This usually means your partner is a big mouth or brags about it and tells everyone what you did. This could ruin your reputation.

Emotionally, it is very important that you trust your boyfriend to treat you the way you want to be treated. You and your boyfriend need to talk about what sex means to you, before sex. Are you guys just playing around, or do you expect a deeper emotional relationship with him because of sex? If you find out after sex that you wanted different things, you will feel rejected, hurt, and disappointed. You need to talk about whether or not you feel ready to handle the emotional consequences that sex can bring to a relationship.

For many girls, if they are sharing themselves sexually, they also want to share a deeper emotional relationship. Sometimes this means an exclusive commitment to only date each other. Sometimes this means seeing each other at lunch at school every day. Sometimes it is talking on the phone every day. Generally, a "deeper intimacy" means an increase in the expectation of some type of communication or contact between the two of you on a regular basis. You may also want to share your feelings about things more deeply, like your feelings toward each other or your experiences in your past. In most cases, emotionally, girls feel they would like to have an increase in intimacy when there is sex involved in the relationship *and* they expect the relationship to be exclusive. You need to discuss this with your potential partner BEFORE sex.

Second, you must trust the guy to respect your privacy regarding sex. A good sexual partner will be discrete (read: keep his mouth shut) about your personal and sexual relationship. If you are not sure if your boyfriend even likes you that much, or if you can trust him, then read Chapter 5 on this subject.

## 6. HAVE MY BOYFRIEND AND I CONSIDERED WHAT WE WOULD DO IF I GOT PREGNANT?

Nearly 1 in 10 teens gets pregnant by the time she is 18. One in five sexually active teens gets pregnant. If you decide to become sexually active, there is a 20% chance that you will get pregnant before you are 20. If you do not practice ANY birth control, there is a 90% chance that you will get pregnant within a year of becoming sexually active (Alanguttmacher.org, 2006).

One of the strangest things that I see as a sex therapist is that very few sexually active teenage girls ever expect that they will get pregnant, even when they aren't using any birth control. Yet, almost none of them want to get pregnant. Somehow they just magically think they won't get pregnant. This is called DENIAL: not facing the truth. If you are thinking of becoming sexually active or you are sexually active, one of the most important things that you and your boyfriend need to consider is how you would handle an unexpected pregnancy. The following information is a guide to your options in this situation, none of which are easy solutions to a difficult problem.

## Four Options for Dealing with an Unexpected Pregnancy

1. Have the baby and keep it to raise yourself.

2. Have the baby and make a plan for adoption.

3. Have the baby and get married or live with the father.

4. Have an abortion.

### Option #1: Keep the Baby

First, your parents or guardians will need to be told or will eventually find out about your pregnancy. For most teenagers, it is a very difficult thing to tell their mother and/or father that they are pregnant.

Just imagine how difficult it might be to tell your parents that you are sexually active. Then imagine telling them that you are pregnant—it's even harder. Nowadays, more and more teenage girls are keeping their children to raise on their own, which is very difficult.

### Real Life Challenges in Teen Parenting

- First, it is very hard to be the only one responsible for caring for the needs of an infant, doing everything all by yourself. Even if you are living with your parents or relatives and they help, there are always conflicts with your parents in how you are raising your child, and the bottom line is that you are the one responsible for this child's health and well-being.
- Second, whether your goals include going to college, finishing high school, or having a career, having a child will interrupt your quest to achieve any goals you have for yourself at this age, or at least it will make achieving them far more difficult because of the responsibilities of parenting.
- Third, financially, most teens will find it hard to care for a child. Although you are entitled to financial support from the baby's father, whether you are married or not, most teens will have to work, apply for welfare or both to pay for the expenses associated with having a child. If you work, there are the problems of balancing the care of an infant with school work, finding daycare, getting transportation, and not spending as much time with your child as you would like.
- Fourth, your life as a teenager as you know it will be over. You will lose most of your freedom when you are tied down to the responsibilities of a baby, not to mention losing sleep!
- Fifth, you may have to share custody of your child. Every biological father has legal parental rights for his child. If he legally requests it, he will get regular visitation or, in some situations, even custody. Even grandparents often have visitation rights.

Often, fathers obtain visitation rights and then leave the child with a female relative of their choice to take care of the child, and he has a right to decide who is around the child on his visitation time. While, in some cases, this may be a blessing, at other times it is a curse. In short, you may be tied to the father of this child and perhaps his family until the child is grown up, interacting with them for 18 years.

## Option #2: Make Plans for Adoption

For many girls, after carrying a baby for nine months, emotionally it is very hard to give up a baby for adoption. The option of adoption, because you are unable to provide a child with the life you want to give him or her, is often a courageous act, and may be the best choice to meet the needs of your child. Unfortunately, some women suffer a sense of loss over their child for years, because of not knowing the whereabouts of their child, how the child is being cared for, wishing they could have raised their child, and just missing their child. Open adoptions can help with these problems of loss, because you know who the child is with and you may obtain pictures and information about the child as he or she grows up. It can be very heartwarming to know your child is well taken care of and you have helped a couple fulfill their dreams of having a family. Yet, in some cases, children who are adopted feel a sense of loss regarding their mother, and they feel rejected or abandoned by their biological parents. Although, in the balance of all thoughts and emotions, an adoption may be the best thing for a mother and child, there are frequently emotional consequences for the father, mother and child.

Also, in many states, a father has legal rights to his child as a parent. Even if you want to make adoption plans for the child, a father has to sign away his legal rights in order for an adoption to occur. In some cases, a father will seek custody of the child, often because his parents or relatives want to have custody. In almost all cases, a father will win custody of his biological child if the alternative is that someone else will adopt the baby.

## Option #3: Get Married

Teenage marriages have a lot of problems and suffer a high divorce rate. Taking care of yourself as a teenager can be very difficult for the most mature and skilled person. It is difficult to get adjusted to taking personal responsibility for all parts of your life on your own. Just think of some of the conflicts you have now with your parents: keeping your room clean, doing your homework, and having money for fun. If you get married, you are suddenly responsible for ALL of these things yourself. On top of this, you will be responsible for an infant's life, too. This is a lot of responsibility for the average teenager. In addition, a lot of teenage relationships do not work out, often because the participants are too immature to know how to treat someone right, fight fairly, and work out problems with good communication. Some teens make it, but they always report that it is a tough life. Many teens now live together, rather than marry, but the same struggles of being a young couple responsible for a young child exist.

You might want to take a look at a couple of movies on being a teen parent. In *Driving in Cars with Boys*, the character Drew Barrymore's character struggles with being a teen parent while trying to get an education. An older movie, *For Keeps*, with Molly Ringwald, shows how hard it is to be young and try to raise a child, even when you are in love.

## Telling Your Parents You're Pregnant— Mary and Bob's Story

**My parents started out their young lives by getting married as teenagers, at 18 and 19, and with my mom being pregnant. Bob and**

Mary loved each other very much and really did think they were right for each other. They were actually engaged nine months to the day when my older brother was born. One of the hardest parts for Mary and Bob in the beginning was telling their parents she was pregnant and that they wanted to get married. Mary went home from college to visit and to talk to her parents about getting married. At first, they just talked in general about her getting married. Her father asked her all kinds of questions like, "Can he support you?" or "Where would you live?" My mother did not know how to answer these questions and knew she just couldn't tell them face to face that she was pregnant and that she wanted to get married. To make things worse, my mother's father was a Baptist minister and my father was Catholic, which was a big problem in the 1950's, sort of like people of different races getting married today. Mary didn't know what to do. She was upset, and she quickly left the house to drive back to school, without even saying goodbye. She left a note on her father's desk, saying, *"If you were pregnant, you'd want to get married, too."*

My grandfather called my mother at school and was calm, asking her to please come back home to let talk to them about it. My grandfather acknowledged to Mary that her mother was emotionally distraught, and he asked Mary to go home for her mother's sake, but he also assured her that they would work it out together. Mary felt guilty because she thought her mother, whom she loved dearly, was probably crying, and she returned home. My grandfather asked my mother one question when she came home: "Do you love him?" Mary answered, "Of course. If I didn't love him, I wouldn't be in this mess."

My mom and dad got married a couple of months later. Initially, my father did not tell his parents that my mother was pregnant. His mother asked him before the wedding, "Do you have to get married?" Bob answered, "No." The truth was, in his mind, that he loved Mary and he *wanted* to marry her. He was not just marrying her because

How Do I Know If I'm Ready for Sex?

**she was pregnant. My dad didn't want his mother to feel her son was being forced into a situation and ruin the wedding for his parents. Bob and Mary didn't tell his parents until she was 6½ months pregnant! She was starting to show! Bob's mother was upset when she found out, not because of the pregnancy, but because she knew Bob knew what she was asking him before the wedding and he had avoided telling her the whole truth.**

My parents did stay together, and they had nine more children. In fact, while they had a few ups and downs, they are still together and happily married today having recently celebrated their 50th wedding anniversary. But again, you need to remember that this is the exception and not the rule for teens who marry, and especially if one is pregnant at the time. Today, 79% (compared to 13% in 1950) of teen mothers are not married when they give birth, although many are living with the father of their child. The obstacles to a successful marriage when the participants are young are simply enormous, but I wanted to show you that success is nevertheless possible, that failure of a teen relationship, even under these difficult circumstances, is not inevitable.

## Option #4: Get an Abortion

An abortion is a medical procedure, early in a pregnancy, to remove a fetus, or a growing "baby," from a woman's uterus before it has grown enough to live on its own outside the womb. Many girls have conflicting feelings about abortion. A lot of guys will pressure girls into having an abortion. One girl's experience with pregnancy and a decision for abortion will be discussed further in Chapter 8 in a story about Cheryl, but for now I want to make the point that you must consider the option of abortion carefully. You must make sure that having an abortion is the right decision for you.

For some girls, there are spiritual considerations as well as emotional considerations in having an abortion. Some girls feel that having an abortion is the same as murder, that is, that an abortion is killing a baby. For some girls, having an abortion is like getting rid of extra cells that do not need to grow in their body, that do not need to grow into a baby. You need to know your view on abortion and/or think it over and/or talk it over with someone.

For some women, there are feelings of guilt and loss that last for years after having an abortion when it is the wrong decision for them, sometimes even if they think it is the right decision at the time of the procedure. Suddenly, when you find yourself pregnant, it is usually a big shock no matter what the circumstances. This means that you should really take some time to get your head back down to earth, so you can search your brain and heart to make the right decision for you. Sometimes talking to a minister or pastor many help you in weighing your options and feelings about abortion, and sometimes, the right decision at the time of the abortion is based on your gut feeling. Regardless, however, you must have someone you can trust to talk to, whether it is a friend, a parent, a doctor, or a counselor. Yet, no matter what anyone else says:

91

> Listen to your own inner voice. Your feelings are your soul's way of talking to you!

## 7. AM I READY TO USE BIRTH CONTROL AND PRACTICE SAFER SEX?

Before having any sexual contact, you need to know how sexual behavior can be risky to your health, and how to protect yourself from these risks as much as possible. Chapter 8 discusses sexually transmitted diseases (STDs) and birth control more fully. While many schools provide some information on STDs and risky sexual behavior, it is important to know how to distinguish unsafe, safer

How Do I Know If I'm Ready for Sex?

and safe sex. Some STDs can kill you, others stay with you for life, and others are painful but will go away with medical attention. You should also be aware that there is really no such thing as absolutely safe sex, and abstinence, used each and every time, is the only sure way not to risk getting a STD. However, you can learn about how to have safer sex.

If you are lucky, you will have or have had a good sex ed class in school. Yet, even the best sex ed courses in high school will not tell you everything about STDs. For example, you can get a STD without having sexual intercourse, such as gonorrhea of the throat or contracting AIDS, from giving oral sex. You can also get genital herpes by receiving oral sex from someone who has a fever blister on or in their mouth. In short, you need to educate yourself thoroughly about birth control and STDs prior to having any sexual contact with another person.

## Do I Know How to Get and Use Condoms to Protect Myself Against STDs?

Condoms can be used to prevent STDs. They do not protect you from every kind of sexually transmitted disease, but they have been proven to help reduce the risk significantly. Condoms can be purchased at drugstores and at some grocery stores. You do not have to be 18 to buy condoms. There are many different types and brands of condoms, which will be discussed in Chapter 8. All it takes is money and a way to get to a store to buy them, or you can go to a health clinic to get free ones. Some people are very shy about buying condoms, or even buying tampons. You must be able to be confident enough to buy condoms to be ready to have sex. Read Chapter Eight for more information on STDs.

## Am I Prepared to Use Birth Control Every Time I Have Sex?

- Do you or your boyfriend know how to get birth control?
- Do we really know what kinds of birth control are available?
- Are you responsible enough to use it every time you have sex?
- Are you responsible in other ways in your life, like with school-work or doing what you're supposed to do everyday, which would indicate that you are mature enough to take birth control seriously as an everyday responsibility?
- Are you willing to take responsibility for birth control yourself and not just count on your boyfriend to take care of it?
- Are you prepared to talk to your parents about getting birth control if you can't take care of your birth control needs for yourself?
- Do you realize that all types of birth control have a failure rate?
- Do you know which type of birth control is the best one for you?

Most girls do NOT want to ask their parents to go to a doctor, because they are afraid to tell them they are sexually active, and realistically, a lot of parents are NOT approachable because they don't want to condone their child's sexually activity. Some girls, once they tell their parents they are sexually active, are afraid their activities will be restricted ("I'll be grounded for life!") and they'll never get out of the house again. For yourself, you need to be realistically sure that you are willing and able to protect yourself from pregnancy by obtaining and using birth control.

## 8. AM I COMFORTABLE ENOUGH WITH MY BOYFRIEND TO TALK ABOUT SEX?

Commonly, many teenage couples are too shy to really talk about sex. However, it is important to have open communication with your partner in order to be ready for sex and avoid getting hurt from sex. Besides asking yourself if you are ready for sex, there are many things you should be able to talk to your boyfriend about before you have a sexual relationship. First, ask yourself if you can talk about other things besides sex. Second, do you feel comfortable and accepted enough by your partner to believe that he will take your opinions and feelings seriously? Do you trust him enough to share your biggest secrets and fears?

*If you can't feel comfortable talking about life in general, you are not ready to talk about sex.*

## Dr. Darcy's Top Teen Talk Topics:

- Do you talk about school?
- Do you talk about your jobs?
- Does he know about your family? Does he understand and/or accept your family situation?
- Does he accept and know your friends?
- Have you talked about your dreams and goals in life?
- Have you talked about your likes and dislikes regarding interests and activities?
- Have you talked about your likes and dislikes about clothing and dress?
- Have you talked about your likes and dislikes about food and going out to eat?
- Have you talked about your likes and dislikes about movies, TV, or books?
- Would you call him when you have a crisis, like if your car breaks down?
- Do you feel like you can talk to him about almost anything, including your values about sex?

- Can you talk to him about how you feel, such as liking him?
- Can you tell him if you like something sexually or not? Like: higher, lower, faster, slower?
- You need to know if either of you is a virgin, if either of you have had other partners, because of the risk of STDs.
- You need to be able to tell your partner when you are having your period.
- Can you ask your boyfriend to wear a condom?
- You should be able to talk about birth control, make decisions about what to use, and decide together to use it.
- You need to talk about the potential consequences of pregnancy.
- Can you agree with each other about having other sexual partners or being "exclusive," meaning you don't date other people or have sex with anyone else?
- Can you feel comfortable saying no?

You can't say yes to sex until you can really say no.

Think long and hard about this statement. This statement is my favorite piece of advice on sex. If you can't say no to sex, then you really aren't confident enough to say yes and mean it! Letting your partner know what you really want from sex, as stated above, is very important for both of you in having positive sexual encounters. Although sexual communication may be embarrassing at first, if you do not have it, there will a lot more problems later. Chapter 6 tells more about how to have good sexual communication, as a foundation of a healthy sexual relationship.

~~~~~~~~~~

> If you can't talk to your boyfriend openly about sex, you are really not ready to have sex!

~~~~~~~~~~

## 9. CAN MY BOYFRIEND AND I "LEGALLY" HAVE SEX?

You need to be concerned with whether or not you and your partner can "legally" have sex, based on your ages. If only one of you is an adult, someone can get in trouble—serious trouble. First of all in, in almost all states, it's against the law and called statutory rape if an adult has sex with a minor, that is, a person under 18. "Statutory rape" means the person having sex has not reached the legal "age of consent" in your state, or is an adult having sex with a minor. For example, in South Carolina and Michigan, the age of consent is 16. This means that it is against the law to have sex with someone who has not yet reached the age of 16. Even if two people love each other, and even if they both say they consented to a sexual relationship, a guy or a girl can get in very serious legal trouble for statutory rape, including being arrested for sexual assault and being labeled a sex offender for life. Most 18 year old guys know what the term 'jailbait' stands for, and you should, too: it means a young girl may be terrifically tempting, but she is too young to have sex with, and he can go to jail if he does.

## The Legal Bottom Line

1. You both have to be the "age of consent' to have a sexual relationship. This age varies from state to state. Call your local sheriff's office and ask about the "age of consent" in your state or country.

2. You both must be minors who are the legal age of consent or you must both be adults.

VIRGIN SEX *for Girls*

96

3. If one of you is a minor and the other is an adult, then it is not legal to have a sexual relationship, and the adult can get into legal trouble, even if you love each other and the minor "consented" to the sexual relationship. If you really love each other, you will both accept the legal reality of this situation, and act responsibly with each other. For example, if a minor gets pregnant, and the father is an adult, he can face legal charges of statutory rape for his actions.

Legal matters aside, age and maturity level can strongly affect your relationship. Most teenagers find that they get along better in a relationship, and especially a sexual relationship, if they are closer in age and maturity level. How close you need to be in age can vary, but generally, two years is a good guideline and three years is pushing it. If you are 14 years old and your boyfriend is 19, eventually you are both likely to find conflicts in this relationship. If you are of different ages, your interests and the activities you engage in may be very different. For example, a 19-year-old may want to go to a bar to see a band, but a 14-year-old can't get into a bar until she is 18 and most parents wouldn't let her go anyway. There may also be sexual conflicts. For example, a 14-year-old girl may be ready for a physical relationship that consists of kissing, hugging, and some touching. A 19-year-old guy may put sexual demands on the 14-year-old that she isn't ready for.

Maturity levels vary a lot among people, regardless of their age. In general, girls tend to be about two years ahead of guys emotionally. As a result, many girls want to date older guys, because emotionally they may relate to each other better. For a 15-year-old girl and 15-year-old guy, some interests may be the same, but they may be very far apart in having an emotional connection. For example, a 15-year-old girl may be want to have deep, intimate conversations

How Do I Know If I'm Ready for Sex?

about feelings, while a 15-year-old guy may still be more interested in playing video games. Having similar maturity levels usually means that you will have more interests in common and you may be more compatible emotionally than not. On the other hand, the older in age that the guy is that you date, it's more likely he will put demands on you for a sexual relationship. Hopefully, with maturity, you can decide together if you are both ready for sex and consider if your can have a sexual relationship without someone getting into trouble legally.

## 10. WOULD I HAVE SEX IF I WEREN'T DRUNK OR HIGH?

Different than the rest of the questions in this quiz, often this question presents itself in a moment, in the moment, when you are in a situation that you are drinking or using drugs. You can make a decision, NOW, to NOT make a decision about sex unless you are sober, and usually this will help prevent many problems. One of the biggest mistakes that teens make, when it comes to sex, is deciding if they are ready for sex when they are drunk or high. It is just simply easier to forget your "conditions" for sex, or to minimize their importance, when you are intoxicated. Most of my clients, both teens and adults, have made at least one sexual mistake, at some point in their lives, because they had too much to drink or, as the song says, "because I got high."

You are much less likely to make good decisions about sex when you are drunk or high. Also, drugs and alcohol can affect your feelings of attraction and intensify your sexual excitement, or bluntly put, can make you feel horny when you normally wouldn't feel that way. Let's say one of your conditions for having a sexual relationship is that you will ALWAYS use a condom until you are engaged or married. When you're drunk, you might decide this condition for sex isn't nearly as important as wanting to be with some really hot guy. Or you may be too high to bother taking the time to go to the place you keep a condom, or remember where it is, to get it in the heat of the moment. One of your conditions for sex might be that you have to have strong attractions to someone before you make out with them. You might find yourself attracted to someone you would never have been attracted to when you were sober, leaving you feeling very embarrassed the next day when everyone finds out who you hooked up with.

> Very often, when people choose to have virgin sex when they are drunk or high, they regret their choices the next day, when they're sober.

You might consent to having sexual experiences or sex for the first time when you are drunk or high, but if you were sober, you would have NEVER had a sexual encounter with that person, or in that place, or at that time. You might just let things happen and not have used your usual good judgment or physical ability to say no. Sometimes, you are just too drunk to care about yourself. Sometimes, people get date raped because they have less ability to avoid a situation or to stop it from happening. Date rape will be discussed further in Chapter 10. Sometimes, people are so intoxicated that they "black out" and do not remember anything of the sexual encounter. Regretfully, one client, named "Shana," remembers nothing of her first sexual experience because she blacked out after drinking excessively. Shana found out that she lost her virginity because there was blood on her sheets when she awoke, and because the guy called her the next day to say thank you for a good time.

If you choose to drink or use drugs, you need to be very careful about the situations in which you put yourself and with whom you hang out. One piece of advice is to have a best friend with you, so you can "watch out" for each other at parties. Parties are terribly dangerous settings for regretful sexual situations. Better yet, stay away from drugs and alcohol in dating situations, especially until you have more experience with both sex and using alcohol. For example, many adults enjoy having one, two or even three beers or cocktails on a Friday or Saturday night. For most people, this is not dangerous drinking behavior. But many adults have gotten drunk once or twice in their lives before they found out their limit in drinking may be only 2 glasses of any type of alcohol, so they learn to stop there. Some people, including teenagers, find they cannot stop when they drink and they have a problem, which will probably require professional assistance. As a teenager, you probably don't know your drinking limits, and it is not a good idea to get into dating situations while you are also experimenting with alcohol.

Make virgin sex sober sex.

# five

# GUYS AND LIES: HOW TO KNOW IF A GUY REALLY LIKES YOU OR JUST WANTS YOU FOR SEX

For most teenagers, friendships, and relationships are the most important things in their life. God, family, school or extra-curricular interests may be very important, but if you are a normal teenager, you think about guys and girls and relationships A LOT. For many teens, friendships, having fun and having relationships are what you think about every day. If you are lucky, you probably have at least one best friend, and hopefully a group of friends, to call, to talk with online, or hang out with. Having friends, whether you are a teen or an adult, is ESSENTIAL. If you don't have friends, you know you need to take a good look at your life and work to make this happen, whether you are popular or a big geek. Yet, having someone like you or even love you (besides your parents or guardians) is probably one of the most significant things in your life.

A lot of teenage guys are not really into having *relationships*. This is not true of all guys: some guys want to have a relationship, with all the elements included, like phone calls, going out, and having an exclusive commitment to someone. However, a lot of guys just want to hang out with their friends, spend time playing sports, make some money working a part-time job, and have a nice car; and they don't really want to be committed to one person. Yet, most of these guys want to have sexual relationships and experiences, too.

On the other hand, most girls do want to have relationships, especially one special relationship with one special person. Most girls only want to have a sexual relationship when it is a part of an exclusive relationship with one special person. This difference between most girls and guys causes a lot of problems.

> The bottom line: Often, most guys are interested in sex first, then maybe a relationship. Often, most girls are interested in a relationship first, then maybe sex.

Generally, girls and guys have very different interests and motivations in getting together. Often, guys are motivated to find a girl who looks great, and then maybe they'll get lucky and have a sexual relationship. Often, a girl's motivation is find someone to like or even to love them, and maybe they'll get lucky and have someone to talk to about all that is important to them. Because of these very different motivations in getting together, a lot of girls get hurt both emotionally and sexually from relationships. Often, girls read a relationship wrong, thinking a guy really cares about them, when it might be that he is mostly interested in having sexual experiences.

It is often very difficult for girls to tell if they can really trust a guy to care about them and not just care about having sex with them. When a girl thinks a guy really cares about her, and then she has a physical relationship with him only to find out that's all he wanted, she feels used and cheap. It is ABSOLUTELY *NOT* TRUE THAT

## ALL GUYS WANT IS ONE THING: TO HAVE SEX, BUT . . .
how do you know if a guy really likes you or just wants you for sex?

## Kaitlyn's Story

Kaitlyn was 17 and had been dating guys for a couple of years. She had had crushes on guys since 6th grade. In middle school, she talked to and was "going with" a few guys, but most of these relationships were short, lasting two weeks to a month. In the beginning of high school, in 9th and 10th grade, she mostly hung out with her girlfriends. She went with one guy in the summer of 10th grade for a couple of months, but it didn't really get serious sexually, not beyond kissing and touching. In 11th grade, she got a huge crush on this guy named Jason. Jason was on the wrestling team, and Kaitlyn started going to a couple of wrestling meets with her friends in order to see him, acting like she merely had a lot of school spirit.

Finally, around Thanksgiving, Jason heard from his friends that Kaitlyn was looking at him and he wanted to talk to her. They didn't have any classes together, which made it kind of hard to get together at first. At a party over Thanksgiving, however, they "met" for the first time. They spent some time talking to each other and exchanged phone numbers. Kaitlyn called him the day after the party. He seemed nice on the phone and agreed to go Christmas shopping with her. She was very excited and liked him more than ever. The day after they went shopping, she called him again, and she asked him to go to the movies with her. At the movies, he started putting some moves on her: they kissed and he tried to feel down her shirt. She felt like he was moving fast, but she really liked him, and he stopped touching her when she moved his hand away from her shirt, so she felt like he respected her. When they were talking after the movie, he said he liked spending time with her, but he told her he wasn't really into calling girls or talking on the phone.

103

Shortly after the movie "date," Kaitlyn's parents went out of town to go Christmas shopping. Kaitlyn called Jason and asked him to come over to her house. Jason hadn't even called her one time, but Kaitlyn didn't really care because he had said he wasn't into talking on the phone, that it just "wasn't him." When Jason came over, he was really making the moves on her. They ended up in her bedroom pretty quickly. When Kaitlyn went to answer the phone in another room, Jason took off all of his clothes and got on her bed. Kaitlyn was pretty surprised when she went back into her room and saw Jason naked, but she was very attracted to him and "he had a great bod!" Kaitlyn felt kind of flattered that he was so bold and undressed, and she thought that he was really interested in her. Jason told her that he really liked her and he wanted to be "her first." Kaitlyn was pretty much blown away by his advances, and she thought that he must really like her and think she is special. She especially felt like he cared about her because he had brought two condoms with him and told her, "I want to make sure that you are protected and you don't get hurt." Although Kaitlyn really didn't know him very well, she really did like him and she thought he was HOT. Kaitlyn thought he really liked her, although he never actually said that.

Kaitlyn decided to go ahead and have sex with him, since it was a good opportunity, with her parents were out of town, and she was able to be alone with Jason. She told him it would be his Christmas present to "give him her virginity." Of course, Jason was happy to accept the gift. Kaitlyn thought everything went really well: Jason was really gentle and moved slow when it came to having sexual intercourse, and she felt OK about it.

After that day, however, Jason avoided Kaitlyn. When she called his house the next day, he wouldn't take her phone call. He wouldn't answer her next five phone calls, either. He avoided her at school, and he actually almost RAN away from her when she saw him in the hall at school. She wrote Jason a note and gave it to a friend to give to him, which he got but never answered. In the letter, she begged him to call her and talk to her, but he never did. Embarrassingly, she went to his house, but he wouldn't come to the door. At his door, his parents told her to leave him alone because he didn't want to talk to her.

Kaitlyn felt embarrassed about trying to get in touch with him, and she decided to give up. She felt like a complete fool. At that point, she began hating Jason. She felt completely used and disgusted with herself. In looking back, she realized Jason did not have any interest in her, except for having sex. She had had such a huge crush on him, that she interpreted every positive thing he said to her as an indication that he liked her. When they were just meeting each other, she thought that maybe he was just the quiet type and that this was why he didn't like talking on the phone. What she realized is that he was just the type to use her and that he really didn't like HER at all.

Kaitlyn felt very hurt, emotionally, by Jason. She really did like him, but she mistakenly assumed that he really liked her back. She read many of the things he did or said as indications that he liked her, when she was actually projecting what she wanted these things to mean. However, although Kaitlyn was partially fooled by herself because she really liked Jason, she was also fooled by Jason. She thought that since he wanted to have sex with her, and be "special" to her, that he really liked her. Kaitlyn fell into a trap that a lot of girls fall into. She really didn't know Jason very well, and she had not spent very much time with him at all. When looking back, she realized that he really didn't show her that he was that interested in her: she had made all the moves to get together, and he just followed her lead. Except for a few nice things that he said which she interpreted incorrectly, he didn't really tell her he liked her or that he was interested in her. What Kaitlyn learned from this was to be much more cautious with guys, even if she really liked them, until she really knew whether or not they were sincerely interested in a serious relationship with her. Unfortunately, she regretted giving her virginity to someone who really didn't care.

Guys and Lies

> A major reason girls regret having sexual relationships is because they feel used or played by a guy.

How do you know if a guy is being genuine or just trying to "get as far" as he can go with you? How are you, as a girl, supposed to know the difference? For starters, it is important to know the difference between just having sex and having a loving, sexual relationship—really "making love." For most people, guys and girls, the difference between having sex and making love is huge. It is sort of like the difference between eating a raw, unpeeled potato and eating a crispy, hot and salted order of French fries dipped in ketchup: the preparation and spices make all the difference. When it comes to sex, caring is the preparation and love is the spice. Adding love to a physical relationship makes it feel different, and it is a difference that most girls want to experience, especially when having first physical and sexual relationships.

Some girls, as discussed in previous chapters, do want to have sex for the first time because of curiosity or because they want to "get it over with." Unfortunately, this often leaves a young woman feeling very unsatisfied, and even emotionally or physically hurt, when it comes to losing her virginity. It is strongly recommended that you engage in initial sexual relationships that are meaningful to you. Remember: you will always remember your first sexual experiences, and they can have an effect on whether or not you actually like sex in the future.

## MAKING LOVE? OR HAVING SEX?

The biggest difference between making love and having sex is how you feel emotionally about your partner. Take the following quiz to ask yourself how you really feel.

# Emotional Quiz: Get Real on How You Feel

1. Is this someone you would choose as a friend?

2. Do you feel "comfortable" with this guy?

3. Do you feel attracted to this guy? Is he hot?

4. Do you fantasize about him? Do you think about him every day?

5. Is this someone you would be proud of being seen with?

6. Do you respect him?

7. Can you express your feelings with him: mad, sad, glad, or scared?

8. Does he seem to have the same attraction and feelings toward you?

9. Do your friends like him?

10. Would you take him home to meet the parents (assuming your parents are sane)?

If you answer "no" to any of the questions, then you might not be emotionally ready for a serious sexual relationship. If you answered "I don't know" or "maybe," then you need to get to know each other better. Listen to your GUT feelings! But you must also remember that, often, if your friends think he is a big loser, you need to pay attention to what they are seeing in him and reexamine your feelings. If you both have loving, caring feelings for each other, it is much more likely that you will be making love, not just having sex.

## Making Love or Having Sex: What Teens Tell You!

Jenna: "Place has a lot to do with it—like if it's in a car or in a bed. Having sex in a car is usually more sport than lovemaking in a bed."

Marcos: "Having sex is just with any girl, but making love is with *my girl*."

Eva: "If it's romantic, then it is making love."

Kathryne: "People talk about caring for each other, like loving or liking each other, when they talk about making love instead of just having lust or horniness for each other."

Mike: "Sportsexing can be a great thing with the right person, but it is not lovemaking." [Sportsexing is having sex outside the context of a relationship]

Rachel: "People call each other very soon, like the next day, after making love. People sometimes avoid each other, at least for a day or week after sex, when it's just "friends with benefits" or with a guy who isn't really interested in you."

Shakisha: "Just because a guy doesn't say he loves you doesn't necessarily mean that he doesn't have deep feelings for you. Some guys just don't talk that way. Guys aren't taught the same way as girls to talk about how they feel."

Katie: "If the person is still there with you in the morning, it's real love."

Josh: "Making love happens way before you ever have sex, and you can see it when you look into each other's eyes. Having sex is like eyes wide shut."

Caryl: "When you kiss or say goodbye at your door and he walks away, notice if he looks back at you or not. If he just walks straight ahead and leaves, he doesn't really care. If he looks back, he's coming back."

# HOW TO KNOW IF A GUY MIGHT BE USING YOU JUST FOR SEX

Too often, girls are fooled into thinking they are really cared for or have a committed relationship with a guy, when in fact, it's a lie. When that happens, and sex is part of the "relationship," girls can get used for sex. Getting played for sex usually makes girls distrust, dislike, and even avoid guys. It can make girls lose their respect for themselves and for the true meaning of sex. Sometimes, girls even blame themselves when this happens, for being naive or stupid, thinking they did something wrong and wishing they could take back the past, which is impossible. Usually when a girl gets used for sex, it is because, in some way, someone lied to her. Even the smartest, most street smart girl or woman can have this happen to them at some point in their lives. The following guidelines are a collection of advice from some of these "played women" who shared their experiences to help you know how to avoid being used for sex.

## 25 Ways You Might Be Getting Played

1.  A guy who just wants sex is not interested in having a real relationship. A real relationship means being friends *and* being friends in front of *his* friends and family. A player doesn't want to meet your friends, and especially not your parents or relatives.

2.  Activities are only or mainly arranged when you can be alone, not in the company of friends or family or going out to do fun things together. A real relationship involves shared activities outside of a bedroom or sexual situation.

3.  He calls you only when it is convenient for him, without considering your needs or wants. Or he leaves you waiting by the phone when he said he would call.

4.  The guy comes over late and drunk, tells you how much he's missed you, says he talked about you all night with his friends

and wants to see you now, at midnight or so. Or he calls and says all these things. Wait to see him when he's sober. Have a relationship based on sober feelings, not with someone who is "drunk and horny" and might say anything to you to get you to have sex with him. If he was thinking about you so much, he would ask you out, not just call you when he's horny.

5. He tells you that you talk too much (unless you really do have a problem with being a big time talker, which you would already know from YOUR family and friends' complaints).

6. When his friends say he talks badly about you, it's true. Even if you confront him and he denies he said those things, believe what his friends tell you.

110

7. He blackmails you. He tells you that he will tell all of his friends if you don't "put out" or "give it up," or he says, "I'll tell them you did it anyway." This behavior is called coercion. It is not loving behavior and it is a warning sign of an abusive personality.

8. He prefers being with his friends instead of you, unless he wants sex.

9. He threatens to drop you as a girlfriend unless you "put out" because he will find someone else who will give him what he wants. This is a sure sign that what he wants is sex . . . not you!

10. When you call him, he is always busy doing something else.

11. He's caught in lies about little things, like where he was last night or why he didn't call. People who lie about little things will lie about big things.

12. If he blames you for his lies, such as saying he was trying to protect you, then run.

13. When you call his house, and there's a girl's voice in the background and he says it's "just some friends" and he refuses to give names, there is an excellent chance that he's cheating.

14. He talks about other girls in a degrading way, like saying nasty sexual things about them (not just noticing a good-looking body). For example, "James" only refers to girls as "whores," not

as women or girls or ladies. If he talks about other girls in these ways, that's the way he sees you, too.

15. If he says demeaning things to you, then says he's "just playing with you" afterwards, he means it and is secretly getting off on it.

16. Is there a long list of ex-girlfriends who still hate him? That "I've changed and realized all my mistakes!" line is believable once, not repeatedly with several girls. A few months after a break up, generally, if a guy was decent to a girl, they can be decent to each other. Hate lasts a long time and is a warning sign.

17. If you've heard that he's got out of town girlfriends, he does. If he goes out of town a lot, then you hear he's got a girlfriend there, he does. If you confront him about it and he says, "No, that's in the past; we're not like that anymore," he's probably lying. "Once a playa, always a playa."

18. When he says he likes to "live for the moment" when you ask about a commitment, your sexual encounter is the "moment" and you shouldn't expect any future encounters of any type. If you feel you have to check up on him, there's probably already a big problem and a reason you feel that way, unless you're a control freak or paranoid. Trust your gut feeling. If your stomach feels like it is being ripped apart, there is a trust problem, and you're probably being used.

19. If a guy gets these sudden urges to just give you attention, but he never has before, see if the urge lasts for more than a day or a two . . . he might just be interested in sex and not interested in you.

20. When guys try to dominate the whole sexual thing, meaning they call all the moves and act controlling, this is a clue that they won't treat you right.

21. If he leaves right after you have sex or big time messing around, you know you got played. A guy who really likes you for more than just sex will also like cuddling, touching, and "pillow talk." This "after sex" may not happen every time you are together, but a good portion of it.

22. If he says, "Don't tell anyone" about our being together, it is a clue that he's a jerk and just wants sex. While you may not want anyone else to know, most guys don't care unless . . . they're embarrassed about you or they have other girlfriends. You know he is just interested in sex if he is too embarrassed to have you as a girlfriend or he wants to play around with other girls.

23. If he is a tease, then don't expect anything other than sex. This is the guy who is just in it for the "chase," not a true relationship or sexual connection with another person.

24. If he flirts excessively with other girls in front of you, that means he doesn't respect you and he is most likely looking around for or hitting on another girl.

25. If he is very untrusting of you, it might be because he is a cheat himself. Watch out for very possessive and controlling guys, meaning they watch your every move or tell you what to do or wear. These types of guys are insecure and sometimes mentally, physically, or sexually abusive to their girlfriends. These guys are looking for a possession to control, not a relationship.

Despite all of these warnings, remember: not all guys are just out for sex. There are a lot of nice guys who can truly care for, love and respect girls, and want meaningful relationships, too. This chapter is to help you avoid bad situations that lead to bad sexual situations that can hurt you for life. If you are looking for a guy who is genuinely interested in you, just pay attention to these warning signs and steer clear!

## GUYS AND LIES AND LINES GUYS USE TO USE YOU

A lot of teens say that "come on lines" are not typically used anymore, but "lines" come in many different forms. Most of the time, guys find that just being nice to girls, talking to them, lying, putting on a show, and supplying alcohol and drugs, such as weed or ecstasy, are enough to make a girl agree to have sex. Sometimes is it just a trick for a guy "to get laid." Again, not all guys are just out to get laid, but this section of the book is about how to know if a guy is using you.

The most common line guys use to attract girls is simply telling them they're cute or attractive. Many girls confuse compliments as a sign of caring. As a teenager, with the unavoidable expectations and conflicts with your parents, teachers, family and friends, compliments are fewer and farther apart than when you were young. Small children just have to be "cute and sweet" to be loved on by the people around them. It is a fact that teenagers are complimented less, criticized more, and touched less by their parents than when they were young children. Girls with a low self-esteem are especially susceptible to reading more into simple compliments, compliments that do not necessarily mean a guy is genuinely interested in them. Words are nice, but they can be cheap. Long lasting actions, like having an ongoing relationship, are more sincere than words alone.

It is almost a given fact that being a teenager means you have low self-esteem and insecurity at times, or that you question your self-image and identity. Part of being a teenager is finding out who you are. When you are unsure of yourself, you often turn to your friends to feel a sense of belonging and acceptance. For girls, this can mean that you are more vulnerable to insincere kindness. Girls are also more vulnerable to apparent kindness and attention from older guys. It can be very flattering at 15 to get attention and feel liked by a 19-year-old or even a 21-year-old guy. The sad truth is that many of the girls who become pregnant every year have adult men as the fathers of their babies. Insincere kindnesses from guys are called lines or come-ons. This section discusses a variety of different lines, with explanations on how to understand and deal with them.

## Lines, Lies, and Comebacks

*"You're so cute and I just want to be with you."*

If he thinks you are so cute and attractive, he will take the time to get to know you, spend time with you, talk to you, meet your friends, meet your parents, and have fun doing things with you before he jumps into just having sex.

*"I'm very attracted to you and I can't help myself."*

If a guy "can't help himself" he has a personal control problem. If he has no patience to really get to know you, except to have sex with you, then he has a mental problem and you need to run away from him. If he can't help himself from wanting to be with you, and if you like him, let him talk to you and get to know you, first.

*"I've got blue balls from not having sex . . .
and I need sex with you."*

You are not responsible for anyone else's sexual needs. Period. First of all, guys get sexually aroused a lot, not just from being with you or from making out. From the time they are born, guys get erections of their penis all day long, about every hour and a half, just from the pure nature of their biology. It is true that if a guy is very sexually aroused and does not have a sexual release, he can get mild soreness in his testicles. This is NOT your responsibility to relieve this for him, however. A guy can endure this short-lived discomfort or he can relieve himself sexually through masturbation. He does not NEED or have to have sex with *you* to survive.

*"Can I come over and use my skills?"*

If the only skills a guy has are sexual play, the relationship is going to get boring very fast. See if the guy has any mental or social skills first. See if he has any skills in talking, having fun, or sharing interests with you. See if he has any imagination regarding how to have fun first, without sex. If that skill isn't there, it won't be there with sex, either.

*"I swear I'll respect you tomorrow."*

If a guy respects you, he will listen to what you want regarding a physical relationship. He will respect your "conditions for sex" and what you are ready for sexually. "Swearing to respect you" is just a line of words. First, learn to trust the guy. Find out it he respects you in other ways before taking the risk of sharing something as private and personal as a sexual relationship or your virginity. Respect is something you and he earn through a relationship that is built on trust and caring, not through words.

*"If you love me, you'll have sex with me."*

If a guy really loves you, he will consider your needs and desires as important as his desire to have a sexual relationship. If he really loves you, he will wait until you are ready for sex. In fact, if a guy *really* loves you, he will be unable to have a sexual relationship with you unless you are truly comfortable and ready, because he will not want to hurt you. If a guy can't put your needs for sex or not to have sex first, he does not love YOU! While he may be truly frustrated that you are not ready for a sexual relationship and he is, if it is true love, he will wait. If he just wants sex, he'll drop you anyway. Some guys will play on your feelings of love to manipulate you into pleasing them. LOVE YOURSELF FIRST!

Guys and Lies

*"If we have sex, I swear I'll treat you the same way after sex."*

On many occasions, guys will try to have sex with a girl, then drop her as soon as sex happens. Sometimes this is because they tried to have sex with you because of the challenge and they like the chase. Once the chase is over, they are off to their next conquest. This is called being used.

In a true relationship, the physical aspect of the relationship is not a black or white thing: like you have a sexual relationship or you don't. The truth is that, in good relationships, the build up to a sexual relationship involves becoming more deeply physically intimate over time. First, there might be talking and holding each other's hands, then there might be kissing. Then there might be hugging, cuddling, and touching. See how you feel with a guy about these types of physical contacts, and pay attention to your responses to them before you continue. Did you like the kissing? Did you feel comfortable with the hugging? At this point, find out if the guy likes you or you like him enough to continue with more personal touching or even sexual touch. See if the guy "acts the same way" after this type of limited physical contact. See if he calls or continues to just want to go out or to hang out with you. The truth or lack thereof in the simple words "I'll be back" should be answered long before a sexual relationship starts.

*"I promise I won't tell anyone."*

Keeping promises is essential to having trust. Trust is built by people making promises and keeping them, whether it is a boyfriend, girlfriend, friend, or parent. It is extremely important when it comes to a sexual relationship that you trust each other. Promises made late at night, perhaps when someone is highly sexually aroused, or even under the influence of alcohol or drugs, can be meaningless.

Trust is made over time. Before you get to the point of having a private, sexual relationship, you should know whether or not you can trust the guy, without his having to give you a line to convince you to trust him. Trust is discovered in easier ways that won't hurt you as much. For example, if you are talking and he says he will call you the next day, does he? Or if you have a date for Friday at 8 p.m., does he keep your date or make excuses? Or did he make it to your house on Wednesday night to help you study? Can he keep a secret or did he tell his friends? These are simple, but effective, ways to find out if you can trust him, beyond words and promises made in the passion of the moment.

## "I love you."

Being in love is often the reason that a couple chooses to have a sexual relationship. After all, sex is often called, "making love." But how do you know if he loves you? Words are not enough. "But, I love you," followed quickly with "So, when can we hook up (for sex)?" is not real love. He has to show you he loves you in non-sexual ways, first, for you to trust his love when it comes to sex. Later in this chapter, you can read about how to know if a guy really likes/loves you.

But then true love is not in and of itself an excuse to have sex if you are not ready. Tina Turner, a famous singer, wrote a song in the 1980s called, "What's Love Got To Do With It?" Listen to this song and you'll hear her belt out the title repeatedly, "What's love got to do, got to do with it? What's love, but a second hand emotion?" Tina Turner was married to a famous singer, named Ike Turner, who physically abused her. Apparently, he loved her very much, but he also beat her senselessly, and eventually, she left him. Even my kids love this "old 80s song" that reveals a universal truth: having love doesn't mean you have to be together or that a relationship will work. Love is not a reason to compromise who you are; it is not a reason to have sex when you are not ready.

Guys and Lies

*"If you don't have sex with me, I'm going to find someone who will."*

At some point in your dating life, whether sooner or later, you will most likely hear this line. Some guys are only willing to be in a relationship if there is sex. Respect his values. Respect your values. If a guy's "condition" for having a relationship, as a teenager, is for it to be sexual, then you might just have different values. This might mean you are simply incompatible, and you need to go separate ways.

This line is often a threat to manipulate your emotions when the person in question knows you like them. Often, when a girl gives in to having sexual intercourse with a guy only because she is afraid she will lose him if she doesn't, the relationship doesn't last. Threats don't make relationships work: true caring and love do. The truth is, if sex is THE most important thing to him, YOU aren't. If that isn't what you want, let him find someone else TO USE.

*"Your outfit really matches my bedspread."*

PLEEEZE . . . this is an example of a really stupid come-on. It is only included here because you need to be prepared for the stupidest things, while trying not to laugh too hard so that you embarrass everyone involved.

*"You're the only one for me."*

It is great to feel special and that you are the "only one" for someone. Sometimes it is true. At that moment in time, you may be the best "ones" for each other. Being special with each other does not mean you have to have a sexual relationship. It means you ACT special toward one another. It means you share intimacy through talking, playing, doing fun things together, doing homework together, raking leaves in the fall, understanding each other's families, *and* through physical intimacy. Intimacy can be created and shared in a variety of ways, until you are ready for sex.

But beware: you might just be the 10th person who has heard that you are "the only one for me" from this guy this year. Some guys try to make you feel like "you're the ONE" to get you to have sex. The "feeling special" button can be powerful, especially when you are a teenager or a young adult. Believe me, there is rarely only one person in this lifetime who is the only person with whom you can have a special relationship and love. And if this is IT, you have a lifetime to make it right, don't you?

### "I just want to talk to you . . . don't go yet."

Sometimes, you are in a situation where you know all he wants to talk about is sex. Appealing to your natural female desire to talk is a great line for a guy. A good come back is: "Call me when you really want to talk." Sometimes this line is just a way for a guy to get you to stay so he can try to weaken your resolve to have sex. Use your intuition and gut feelings: if the date has turned into a pressured situation for physical intimacy and/or sex and you need to get out of there: GO. You can always talk over hamburgers at McDonald's tomorrow at noon.

### "I think I love you, but I won't know until I have sex with you."

Interpretation: Obviously this guy doesn't know the difference between love and being horny. If he doesn't love you before sex, why do you want to make love? Or how could the two of you make love if he doesn't know if he loves you? Tell him to talk to you sometime when he has grown up and knows his own feelings.

*"If we use a condom, you are still a virgin."*

Some girls really don't know the definition of "virginity." A girl's virginity is usually something special to her. Some guys try to convince girls that if they are wearing a condom (or you do it standing up, or if he just puts it in for a second, or if he doesn't ejaculate, etc.), then that sex "doesn't count against being a virgin." Technically, losing your virginity means a penis enters your vagina. It doesn't matter if he is wearing a condom or not, if he ejaculates or not, or how long it lasts. If a penis penetrates your vagina, you are no longer a virgin. See Chapter 7, on Real Sex Ed: The Sexual Dictionary, for more information on virgin sex.

*"I'm a virgin, and I want to lose my virginity to you because you are so special."*

First of all, guys often lie about their virginity (and so do girls). IF you believe this and don't just take it as a come on, enjoy the flattery. Be glad that he thinks losing his virginity is special. It should be special to both of you. However, if the situation is so special, you both want to make sure it is the right time. If he thinks you are so special, then he will wait until you are ready and both of you can comfortably and responsibly share a sexual relationship.

*"Let me put it in just one time."*

This line refers to the guy who asks to just put his penis inside of your vagina one time and quickly get out. This line is generally a lie, even with guys who have the best of intentions. Once there is sexual penetration, most guys do not and will not stop, or at the very least will beg for more. Do not be fooled by this or get yourself into this situation. If you don't want to have sex, then just say "NO," because "putting it in just one time" may well lead to his penis remaining inside you until he is finished.

*"I'm not a virgin: I'm experienced and it'll be good."*

First, you do not have to be experienced to have a very positive sexual experience. Two virgins on their wedding night can have the most wonderful sexual experience together. Second, no matter how experienced he is, sex with him won't be good unless you are ready, mentally and physically, for sex. The time must be right for you. No sexually experienced person can make you ready for sex. Before you have virgin sex, know yourself: what you want is much more important than your partner's experience. The best sexual experience is most likely to happen when you develop a sexual voice about who YOU are and what YOU want, and this is true whether we are talking about kissing, touching, or something more.

121

> You are the major ingredient in having a positive sexual experience, not someone else.

Besides, even if a guy has had sex 100 times, this doesn't guarantee he'll be a great lover. He may not have known what he was doing all 100 times and still doesn't. Many adult, married men don't know what they are doing, either. Making love is an interactive activity, which means you learn from and listen to each other. Some people have that capacity without ever having sex with someone, and some people never develop this ability, no matter how many sexual experiences they have had.

*"Nobody will know, so it won't matter."*

First, go back to the trust issue. You have to know if you can trust someone to be private about your sexual relationship. This is not

Guys and Lies

dependent on words; it is dependent on the trust you have in a relationship that is learned and earned *over time*.

Second, YOU will know. It does matter. It matters to YOU. You will live with your decision for the rest of your life. YOU need to do what matters to YOU. If you're a virgin and your thoughts and feelings on when and where and with whom doesn't matter to this person, then YOU aren't very important to him either and you're being used.

### "C'mon, everyone's doing it."

No, NOT everyone is doing it. Only 53% of high school girls have sex before graduation, and many of those who have had sexual experiences regret it. Some don't regret it, but many will tell you they have had sex when they actually haven't and many who have had sex will tell you they enjoyed it when they did not. So, even if your friends all tell you they have "done it" and loved it, don't necessarily believe it. People lie to fit in. But even if you know for a fact that every single one of your friends has had sex and you are the lone virgin in your crowd, this is not a good reason to have sex. This line is peer pressure at its worst. If someone has to pressure you into having sex, it is highly likely that you really don't want to do it. Believe it or not, when many people are ready for sex, they WANT to do it, and they don't have to do it because other people are doing it.

### "Just this once . . . I won't ask anymore"

And the sun won't come up tomorrow, right?

### "I'm going away (to school, the army, vacation, etc.) And this will be our only chance."

If this is your only chance to be together and you truly love each other, you may be choosing to have a very special sexual experi-

122

ence with a person you love. Virgin sex should always be a special, memorable occasion, but do not fool yourself into believing that having a sexual relationship will keep you together. If you or your partner are in the middle of major life changes, it is likely that you may never see each other again or cross paths to have a relationship again; and even if you do, who is to say that one or both of you will not have changed and therefore you won't feel the same way about each other after some time apart. Read about special occasion sex in Chapter 4. Remember, you may love to enjoy each other's company and have fun in other, memorable ways than having sex together.

"Special occasion" sex can be a type of pressure you are likely to encounter in your dating years (and beyond). You may choose to enjoy a special occasion by sharing a sexual experience. However, there is a certain amount of coercion in this line, using guilt to make someone do something they don't want to, or are not ready to, do. Do you want to have a sexual experience out of guilt or obligation? Let's get back to the basics: a sexual relationship is about expressing and sharing love. Guilt and obligation have no place in love, especially as a reason for a first sexual experience.

You might want to review this section by yourself, or better yet, with a best friend. Come up with your own "lines" and possible responses to guys who use them. You and your friends have your own unique "lingo," or way of saying things. Instead of being surprised or caught off guard with a guy, having lost the gift of speech to the butterflies in your stomach and not knowing what to do, think of your own comebacks. Think on your own, or with your friends, of what you might say in advance and how to say it in your own way in order to prepare yourself for the situation when it arises. This can be a fun game to play with your girlfriends on a weekend sleepover. Even if this section appears to be geeky or old fashioned, it can at least start a good conversation and make you laugh.

### How Do You Know If a Guy Really Likes You?

It is truly important to know if a guy really likes or loves you or if you are being used, especially just for sex. I wish I could give you a guarantee that you will know the difference, but no one can. Short of giving you a foolproof test to make sure you are not being used, however, I will give you a guide to follow to at least increase the odds that you will know one way or the other. With the help of many teenage clients and my own teenage children, we tried to put together a long list of guidelines to help you figure out if a guy is being honest with you and truly cares about you. Remember, you want to know if someone really likes or loves you BEFORE you have any intimate or sexual relationship at any point in your life, but this is even more true when the time comes for you to have virgin sex.

124

## The Real Thing

- He has time in his life for *you*.

- He makes an effort to see you at school or at work (if you go the same school or work together).

- He tells you he likes/loves you. **He has to tell you directly.** Don't assume anything. Don't read into anything else he does or says. But remember, even if he tells you that he cares for you, he may not be sincere. The point here, *for starters, is that you must not "read" meaning into his behavior that is not there. He has to at least tell you that he cares about you. Period. Then you must decide whether or not you can trust him enough to believe what he is saying.*

- He shows affection toward you in front of his friends.

- **He calls you** regularly just to talk, not just to hook up for sex.

- He gives you some things with sentimental value attached to them for him, for example, a class ring, a favorite necklace or a favorite t-shirt to wear.
- He'll call you just to hang out, and every hang-out session doesn't involve sexual pressure or making moves on you.
- He will let you drive his car.
- He calls you by your name to your face a lot.
- He approaches you in the hallway at school.
- He sits next to you in class.
- He is there for you at times of crisis: he'll stay up all night with you just to study for a horrible exam, if only to get ice for your Dr. Pepper and rub your back. He goes to the hospital with you when your grandmother is sick.
- He makes an effort to spend time with you. The relationship does not just consist of you making the effort or the plans to get together.
- Sometimes he pays for dates, not just split pay or you pay.
- He invites you to his home.
- He calls you a friend as well as a girlfriend.
- He holds you when you cry.
- He treats your friends with respect.
- He likes it when you make the moves on him.
- He will be affectionate in public, not just behind closed doors.
- The amount of non-sexual affection privately and publicly should be the same. For example, he will give you just as tight a hug in front of other people as he does when you're alone.

- He remembers birthdays and important anniversaries or holidays with a thoughtful, although not necessarily expensive, gift.

- He will introduce you to his family.

- He talks to his parents about you. You know this when you meet his parents and they know some things about you already.

- He stops when you say stop, no matter what is happening or why you want to go no further.

- He wants to have a real relationship with you. A real relationship includes trust, which means he does what he says he is going to do to the best of his ability.

- He gives you little thoughtful gifts for no reason that have special meanings for you. For example, he gives you a pair of kitty cat earrings because you love cats.

- He calls you or contacts you very soon after you have been physically close, like big time making out, just because he is thinking about you.

- He will watch out for you when you are drinking and not want you to get drunk.

- You feel **comfortable** with him. You are not always wondering what is going on in this relationship.

- He is as affectionate with you when he is sober as when he has been drinking.

- He makes an effort to see you when you are really needing to see him.

- He writes you a note, e-mail or card expressing his feelings.

- Basically, he is always being a good friend. If a guy isn't a good friend outside the bedroom, he'll make a lousy friend, eventually, inside the bedroom, even if he is really nice at first.

- He knows how to express feelings of love through conversation, not just by saying "I love you." He asks about your day, for example.
- You do things together and develop or share interests. This is beyond simply watching videos, but rather it includes activities like throwing a Frisbee around or painting clouds on the ceiling of your bathroom.
- He cares about and asks about your schoolwork, work or activities.
- He shows up at events that are important to you, like your sports games or your grandmother's birthday party.

Hopefully, if you can figure out if a guy really likes you, you will be more likely to make better decisions about having a relationship with him, especially a sexual relationship. Once you've figured out whether or not he likes you, you need to figure out if he is likely to treat you right. Again, there are no guarantees that, even if a guy likes you, he will be the right person for you. So, I've put together a mini personality test for you to check out your guy's potential for treating you right and not taking advantage of you or hurting you in an emotional or sexual way. Psychologically, people are very similar in the way they act in one situation and how they will react in another. So, it is important to know what kind of person someone is, so you can predict what kind of person they might be when it comes to important things, like relationships, love, and especially sex.

How a guy treats you in a relationship will be the same way he will treat you sexually.

If a guy is loving, caring, and pays attention to you when you are going out for a date, he will be loving, caring, and attentive when it comes to kissing and touching you. If a guy is really into himself, how he looks for example, checking himself out in the mirror more than you do, or spending more time making plans with his friends, he is going to be into himself and selfish when it comes to a physical relationship with you, too. If he's into pleasing himself first in life, he'll be interested in pleasing himself first in sex, too.

> You really don't have to have sex with a guy to know what it would be like to have sex with him.

To help you figure out what kind of personality a guy has, I have developed two easy personality tests that do not require years of education, expensive testing devices, or a psychologist for you to get a clue as to what a guy is really like, both in his personality and as a lover.

## Dr. Darcy's Quick Personality Test for Guys

IMPORTANT: WRITE out your answers to the following questions BEFORE you read the answer key below.

1. How does your boyfriend drive? Is he cautious and careful? Is he a little adventurous but follows the rules? Does he get mad when someone cuts him off, or does he let it roll off his back? Is he patient in traffic, making the best use of his time, using conversation or music to distract him, or does he have road rage? Does he keep his car nice looking or is it sort of trashy? Is he kind to other drivers, like letting them into traffic; or is he impatient, riding the bumper of the guy in front of

VIRGIN SEX *for Girls*

him? Is his middle finger his major source of communication with other drivers?

2. How does your boyfriend treat waitresses (or fast food clerks)? Is he courteous? Is he patient when the restaurant is obviously busy or does he complain? Is he generous with a tip or stingy? Does he appreciate the service or criticize every flaw to avoid paying a tip? Does he treat the server like a slave? Is he complimentary or degrading? Is he basically understanding or basically angry when mistakes happen?

SCORING: Underline the adjectives and adverbs or descriptive words in your answers to the above questions. STOP. Do that now before reading any further.

These are the descriptive words that apply to your boyfriend. These descriptive words are the same ones that apply to how a boyfriend will treat you on an emotional and intimate basis, *including a sexual relationship*. Think about what you want and make a decision that you deserve to be treated right, especially when it comes to having a sexual relationship. How he treats other people is how he will eventually treat you, even if he acts really nice and is a perfect gentleman to you at first. That is, his real personality will show through in other situations like those in the test.

# six

# THE BEGINNING OF SEX

People are sexual beings from before the time they are born. However, most parents do not think about their children as sexual beings even when the children reach their teens. William Masters was the "father of sex therapy," and he became interested in sex as a field of study when he was a medical intern delivering babies in the 1950s. Dr. Masters was surprised to see that some male babies were born with erect penises. He was quite surprised and asked the doctor in charge if that had ever happened before. The doctor told him no, that it was just an unusual thing. But Dr. Masters found out, after attending many births, that it was a COMMON happening! This motivated Dr. Masters to become interested in the study of sex. Later, he found out that male babies get erections even before they are born, when they are developing in their mother's wombs. This means that babies are sexual beings from before birth! Later, Dr. Masters found out that girls were wired sexually at least from birth because infant girls have lubrication or wetness in their vaginas! So many times, adults expect that their kids should "save sex for marriage" and not have sexual feelings, thoughts or behaviors until they are adults or married, but people have sexual feelings from the very beginning of their lives.

*You are wired for sex from birth, and it's normal.*

## FIRST SEXUAL FEELINGS

People are often curious about when they begin to have sexual feelings. A common question is, "When do people begin to masturbate?" The answer I give is: "When their diaper comes off." Often, this is in the bathtub prior to a baby's potty training. Babies stretch their arms out all around them: in the air, on the bath toy, in their eyes, on their toes, and at some point, they touch their genitals. They realize this feels GOOD. So they touch themselves again and again. Some parents react by moving their baby's hands off their genitals because they perceive self-touch to be "BAD" or "DIRTY." First of all, the baby is in the bath . . . how can it be dirty? But why is self touching bad? Because it is babies who are touching themselves? YES, that is, according to many parents. They simply do not think that a child should have sexual awareness of even a rudimentary sort, like touching him or herself. This is where the "Sex is BAD" message starts. Parents move their baby's hands away because their hand is in the "wrong place." The result is that this place, the child's own genital area, is perceived as wrong by the child from infancy, in spite of the fact that sexual feelings are natural and begin even before a child is born. But to some parents, genital touch, let alone actual sexual behavior, is suddenly supposed to be right only after the rite of marriage right?

In our society, what is important about sex is that sexual feelings are private and sexual actions are private. Our culture holds that children need to be taught about being private with all forms of sexual touch. It is not uncommon for a three year old who is potty trained and diaper-free to sit in front of the TV and touch or rub on his or her genitals, unconscious of the fact that they are even doing so. They are sitting there with their "blankie" in one hand and sucking on their

131

The Beginning of Sex

thumb or fingers, and the other hand is touching their genitals for pleasure or comfort. Or a 3 year-old boy runs around the house laughing, using his penis as a rudder, pointing it in every direction he wants to go. It is upsetting for some parents to have a child openly masturbate or be naked. At this time, because of how our culture feels about the practice, a child needs to be taught about privacy and being discrete, like telling him or her to only touch their privates in their room or bathroom, when they're alone. Unfortunately, this isn't what usually happens: a child is often told to "stop touching yourself down there" or "that's dirty." This is the beginning of sex, when a child is told again that sexual touch or pleasuring is bad or dirty or wrong, which is the beginning of the association of shame with sex.

A big problem in our society is that many children are taught from the beginning of their lives that even nudity, let alone the natural sexual functioning of their bodies, is WRONG. For a lot of you teenagers reading this book, you may have one or more memories of being told that nudity or touching yourself is wrong. Often there is no gentle guidance in teaching you PRIVACY, only the lessons of SHAME, rather than lessons on the wonders of what God invented: Sex.

## Darleen's Story

Darleen was about 8 years old when she was in the tub bathing herself. By this age, she could wash her own hair and take a bath by herself. One time, she took the hand held showerhead massager and used it to wash her privates. She found out that this felt good and she liked it. One day, her mother walked into the bathroom and saw what she was doing and started screaming at her. As Darleen remembers it, her mother grabbed the shower massager violently out of her hand, then told her she was bad and that what she was doing was bad and to never do it again. Then she got yanked out of the tub and sent to bed.

Darleen felt very scared and uncomfortable about sexual touch

**after that incident. She NEVER talked to her mother about sex, even as a teenager and afterward. Darleen's mother never talked to her about sex, except to say, "All guys want is sex and it isn't worth it, so don't do it." Darleen became a little rebellious as a teenager and went out on her own to find out about sex. She became somewhat sexually promiscuous (having casual sex), and she had several negative experiences with guys. It wasn't until much later that she learned through positive experiences what sexuality was really all about.**

Sometimes parents teach children that sex is bad or wrong by the way they react to sex and/or simply by not talking about it. Children learn that if things are kept secret or hush-hush, something must be wrong or bad. Parents teach shame by getting embarrassed when a sexual topic is brought up in a conversation or in a movie or on TV. In fact, parents can teach you to be uncomfortable about sex just by getting all red-faced and uncomfortable with the subject of sex. As a teen, you need to realize, even if you haven't had this message from the very beginning of your life, that sexual feelings are normal. Nudity and sex are totally natural and wonderful, and some people believe these things are a gift from God.

## AFFECTION

Sharing affection is a natural expression of human feelings between two people. Most teens have crushes and feelings of attraction toward others. However, many teens are shy about sharing affection because of the way our society and our families teach us to be awkward or ashamed about it. One way that parents teach shame about affection is by not showing their love for each other openly in front of their children.

As a couple, my husband and I have openly danced, kissed, and hugged each other in front of our children. It is so sad, but even by the age of 8 our kids were saying, "OH, GROSS, there you

133

go again" or "Get a room." I'm not talking about a tongue lashing with hands roving all over the body. I'm talking about a brief kiss when we greet each other or a dance to the radio on a Saturday morning. Isn't it sad and pathetic that simple gestures of sharing love are seen as unusual or GROSS? In truth, our children have said they like us loving each other and being affectionate . . . but they say that we're WEIRD compared to their parent's friends. IT'S OK, BUT WE'RE WEIRD.

Isn't it weird that sharing affection is seen as weird?

How are you expected to have normal feelings, such as liking and lusting after each other, and feeling affection or loving someone, as you get older? How can you be expected to get to adolescence without sexual inhibitions and "hang-ups?" When parents show or tell their kids that affection, love, and sex are bad, how can they possibly have GOOD SEXUAL RELATIONSHIPS?

Attractions and affection toward other people are natural.

Learning how to feel attraction and express it positively is what you need in order to realize this fact.

## BODY IMAGE: GETTING COMFORTABLE WITH YOUR BODY

### Body Image Problems—Shari's Story

Shari had a body image problem from the age of 13. Shari's mother would continually walk in on her while she was taking a shower and make negative comments about her body, like, "Your butt is getting a little pudgy" (she was a size 5 in jeans), or "Don't forget to wash your privates or they'll smell at this age." This made Shari feel like she was fat or that her body had a bad odor others could detect and she couldn't. Shari's father also made her feel uncomfortable with herself. When she had gained 10 pounds or so in high school, he said to her, "You'll never get dates if you are fat." Shari felt very self-conscious and uncomfortable with her body.

Later, when Shari was seriously dating, she did not want to be seen nude with the lights on or have oral sex. With oral sex, she feared the guy would think her vagina "smelled" bad and she would turn him off. Shari hated her body and began to diet and exercise constantly, so she would be "acceptable." She developed an eating disorder and almost died from being too thin. By the time she was 27, she had never had a long-term relationship with a man, as she was too self-conscious and ashamed of her body to get close to someone.

Body image is a huge, huge problem with teens's feelings about their sexuality, especially girls. Most teens think they are too fat, too skinny, or their butt is too big. They think that their breasts are too small or they have some other negative feelings about their body. Your feelings about your body will affect your feelings about your sexuality. Also, a bad body image can lead to serious problems like eating disorders, depression, and even "cutting," which is making cuts with a sharp object on one's body.

A good body image starts at home. It starts with parents feeling comfortable with themselves and with nudity generally, even if they are only comfortable with these things to a limited extent, so their children don't grow up feeling ashamed about themselves. A lot of teen girls tell me that they have never seen their mother change clothes or even change in a locker room. This can give girls a message of being ashamed of nudity or that there is something otherwise wrong with it. The lack of comfort with changing clothing, for example, can make teens feel the same way about their own bodies—uncomfortable. If your parents feel relaxed about their bodies, chances are, you will too.

## Uncomfortable with Her Body—Clelia's Story

Clelia never felt comfortable with her body, not for many years at least, and this continued into her early 30's. Her mother was always very intrusive, which means she lacked a sense of privacy when it came to interacting with Clelia, even regarding her body. Clelia's mother was very controlling and judgmental in other ways, including her behavior, her dress, her friends, her speech, and her activities. Her mother came from a rich, upper-class life, and she had specific ideas about how her daughter should look and act. It was not very easy for Clelia to feel comfortable with life in general. Clelia always felt bad about herself growing up, because she always felt like she was doing something wrong, according to her mother's standards.

One example of her mother being controlling and intrusive was when Clelia had a period. Clelia used tampons, and she found out that her mother counted the number of tampons she used each menstrual cycle! Clelia felt like she had been personally violated by her mother. She felt like she couldn't even have a normal body function, like a period, without her mother watching over it. This led Clelia to feel uneasy and uncomfortable about her body and natural sexual functioning.

As an adult, Clelia still had problems with feeling comfortable with her body. She often felt fat and unattractive when she was naked. Even when she got married, she couldn't feel comfortable being naked with her husband, and that sad fact ruined her sexual relationship with him. It didn't help that he was just as critical and mean to her as her mother had been to her. After years of therapy and reading lots of self help books, Clelia got a divorce and decided to learn how to accept herself and figure out what made her happy. It

**was not until Clelia's second marriage, when she was 38 years old, that she felt loved and accepted, and she finally learned to accept her body and to enjoy nudity.**

As was the case with Clelia, your parents can have a big part in making you feel uncomfortable about your body. Sometimes your parent's problems or hang-ups don't have anything to do with body image, but if you don't feel good about yourself in general, you may focus your negative perceptions on your body when you feel badly about yourself. Try to separate your feelings from your parents' opinions if they have a problem with sexuality and nudity or body image, and be realistic with yourself. This is hard to do if their views on these subjects are the only thing you know. If you really have a problem with your body, talk to your friends, other relatives or even your doctor; but make sure that the person you choose is reliable and not someone with hang-ups of their own regarding these subjects. Try to get a reliable and objective outside opinion to help you achieve a realistic view of yourself.

If a reliable outside opinion confirms your worst fears—that you have a few pounds (or 50) to lose or you're a bit out of shape—do something right about it. Go to the basics: eat right and exercise. Regular exercise is the number one way to look your best and to feel good, too. If you are seriously overweight, you should talk to a doctor about it. If you are merely 5–10 pounds "overweight," like almost all teen girls in American think they are, you need to work on getting more comfortable with your body. One way to do this, besides exercise and healthy eating, is by talking to yourself. You need to have a loving, accepting attitude toward your body. Seek out your good features and compliment them. Do not look in the mirror and make hateful criticisms to yourself on a regular basis: this will only hurt you. Girls and guys like it when you are relaxed and happy with your body. Almost all guys would rather date a girl who weighs 170 pounds and feels happy and sexy about herself than a 107 pound girl who won't eat, won't let him look at her even in a bathing suit let alone when she is naked, and complains about being fat.

Having a good body image may start at home, but our society, in general, has problems with body image and nudity. On TV, in movies, and in magazines, our culture is obsessed with thinness and having a "perfect body." It is hard not to compare yourself to models and actresses who seem to look perfect and fulfill our culture's unrealistic idea of beauty. Of course, many of these people are not natural and their look has been changed by plastic surgery. Also, most magazines alter pictures, with the help of the computer, and consequently the pictures are fake. For example, one common camera trick is for women to tape up their breasts with duct tape in order to make them look bigger (and the tape is painful to remove, by the way). It is very hard for girls and women to remember that most media images aren't real and to accept that they themselves are beautiful and perfect just the way they are, the way nature intended.

Some people think that a body image problem is an American thing—that we are just SO hung up on body image. They may be right. For example, I think that foreign countries that allow nude sunbathing have a lot to teach Americans. One of the great things on nude or partially nude beaches is that you see ALL kinds of bodies: big and small bodies, bodies with scars and freckles, big boobs and no boobs, flat tummies and fat tummies. In Greece, I saw that most people, even the 300-pound 50-year-old woman and the 80-year-old man in a bikini bathing suit, looked comfortable with themselves. Although this may sound gross to you, it is just people feeling comfortable with what nature has given them. So many, many teenage girls, and even some guys, are so freaked about their bodies that plastic surgeons are multimillionaires all over this country. In America, you have to work at being comfortable and happy with your body.

## SEXUAL COMMUNICATION

Part of the beginning of sex is sexual communication. Honestly, it is astounding to me how many teens actually do have sex before they are able to even talk about sex! No, it is not a requirement to be able to talk about sex before you actually have sex, because many girls have done it and even many grown women do it! Remember the story of Suzanna from Chapter One? Suzanna would just put her hands over her face and the boys would "do the rest." Suzanna got pregnant, dropped out of high school, got married at 15, and had her second child when she was 17. Suzanna got NOTHING out of sex: No physical, emotional, or sexual pleasure. She was looking for love, but never felt loved because she never talked to the guys about her feelings or even her sexual thoughts or feelings. She never spoke up to say what she wanted or didn't want sexually, including using birth control. She simply covered her eyes with her hands and let the boys have sex with her. Sex wasn't for her or about sharing love or even having sexual pleasure, it was about her trying to get a guy to like her, love her, and pay her attention. Not surprisingly, after she was married, at only 17, she didn't like sex. How could she? Suzanna's feelings, thoughts, desires, values and needs weren't a part of the sex she experienced. In therapy, Suzanna began to explore how she really felt about sex, for herself, first. Then, she learned to speak up, ask for what she wanted and didn't want, and say specifically how she wanted things to be sexually. Only then did Suzanna begin to enjoy making love with her husband. And guess what? He started to like sex more, too! Sex begins with exploring what is right for you, so *you* can be a part of sex, from the beginning.

> Sex begins with experiencing your own thoughts, ideas, and values about sex for yourself, first. Sex with another person begins with communicating and sharing your ideas, values, and feelings about sex, before you ever have a physical relationship together.

In Chapter 4, one of the questions in the quiz "Are You Ready for Sex?" asked whether or not you can talk to your boyfriend about sex. Sexual communication is essential before you are ready for a safe and healthy sexual relationship. Sexual communication means you can talk about sexual topics, including sharing your values, feelings, thoughts, ideas, as well as your likes and dislikes about sex. First, you start with exploring what is right for you as an individual. Then, you begin to develop a sexual voice, which means speaking up about what you want or don't want sexually, or in the beginning, what you think you think about sex. The next step is to share your thoughts and feelings about sex with your sexual partner, which is often difficult at first, for most people. Sex is a private matter and sharing and disclosing your feelings, at first, is personal. People often feel shy and vulnerable when sharing their sexual thoughts and feelings. People are afraid that someone will make fun of them or ridicule them. Learning to open up and discuss sexual topics is essential for the beginning of sex, and as a foundation for healthy sexuality for life.

Here are first steps, beginning steps for learning and practicing sexual communication.

## Dr. Darcy's Secret Three Step Solution for Sexual Communication

A. Talking and Listening
B. Self Disclosure + Acceptance = Closeness
C. Disclosing/discussing sexual topics

A.

Communication starts with simply talking and listening. Most girls like to talk and are pretty good at it, but you might need to learn to listen better with guys, and make sure they listen to you, too! Pay attention. Does he pay attention to you? Do you feel a genuine sense of caring about what you say? If you don't feel it, you're talking to the wrong person. Move on. Try again. Try using "Dr. Darcy's Top Teen Talk Topics" in Chapter Four, to get your conversations started. Just practice basic communication first, before you move on to sexual communication.

B.

*Self disclosure* is sharing something personal, *accepting* is how one responds to it, and *closeness* will follow. First start with self-disclosure, which means you tell something personal about yourself. At first, you might start with something simple about yourself, like your favorite color, favorite food, or who is your best friend. Then, if you feel comfortable and accepted, move on to more personal things, like your last boyfriend, or even family problems. Second, people wait to see how someone responds to what they tell about themselves. If someone acts accepting, or likes what you are talking about, you feel more comfortable and you can feel closer to that person. If someone acts indifferent, doesn't care, or is not accepting, it may make you feel distant (or want to be), instead of feeling close, right?

When you know that someone is listening and being accepting, you are more likely to talk about personal things that are important to you. When two people share personal thoughts and secrets and experiences, they become friends and sometimes more. Sometimes, people start feeling attractions to each other. When you feel close attractions and you can talk about "everything," you might begin to feel comfortable to move on to talk about sexual topics, too.

C.

Sexual communication is a lot like regular communication: it uses the same formula:

Self Disclosure + Acceptance = Closeness.

The same formula of talking, listening, and being accepted add up to closeness, except with sexual communication, you add in sexual thoughts and feelings to the conversation. In simple terms, when you talk openly about sex, and you both act accepting, caring, and supportive, then you will feel close and more intimate with each other, sexually speaking.

One of the ways you might want to talk about sex as a couple, when you feel like you are comfortable and close enough, is take the "Dr. Darcy's Am I Ready for Sex?" quiz in Chapter 5, together. Whether you are a virgin or you've already had sexual experiences, it's important that you are ready to sexually communicate for any new sexual experience, whether you are 16 years old or 61 years old! As a girl, you really do need to learn to talk to guys about sex, from the beginning of your sexual life and beyond, each and every time. The beginning of sex means using your sexual voice, sharing your sexual thoughts and feelings, and feeling comfortable with sexual communication before you move on to sharing sexual behaviors.

## FROM THE BEGINNING OF SEX TO THE NEXT SEXUAL BEGINNING

Sexual communication is not a one time event! Some people think sexual communication is when you have "THE sex talk" and believe "Whew! We talked about STDs, birth control, and what we want to try sexually, GREAT! Now we got THAT over with and we can have sex!" WRONG! Sexual communication is the beginning that brings you from how you feel from the start, to the next starting place, depending on how you experience individual sexual situations.

At first, when you are exploring your sexual self, you think you think something about sex. Yet, when you experience a sexual situation with someone, you might find out that you don't think what you thought after all. Something as simple as the first sweet experience of kissing someone might not turn out as you planned. Let's say you have talked to this guy, had a huge crush on him, saw him every day, and plotted ways to be alone with him for weeks. The moment came when you got together, and you hugged and kissed and . . . it felt like you were kissing a frog! Seriously! This can happen! You just don't know how you are going to feel about a person, a situation, or a kiss, until it happens. When it happens to feel wrong, then you have to deal with it. You have to communicate how you really feel or you'll be betraying yourself, and them, if you go along with something that doesn't feel right. You have to tell someone the chemistry, the magic, the attraction was not there, as you thought it would be, and you changed your mind.

Can you imagine how hard it is to tell someone that you didn't like kissing them? It's embarrassing, you don't want to hurt someone's feelings, and you have to figure out an escape plan and fast. Honestly, honesty is the best policy, by saying something like "I'm sorry, but the feeling just isn't there for me." The truth is, if it isn't there for you, chances are good that they aren't feeling it, either. However, since people try not to hurt each other's feelings, they may even tell little white lies to make excuses to escape, like saying they have to go home to get their homework done or feed the cat. Even if you communicate indirectly, by making lame excuses, you know you have to let the other person know you changed your mind.

Now, rather than a sweet first kiss, let's say you are experiencing sex for the first time with someone. Sex is more personal. Sex is more serious. Sex is more naked, physically and emotionally. You've had the first kiss, the second kiss, and the 100th kiss with a great guy and the chemistry is there, for real! You've moved on from making out to wanting to make love. You do all the right things: you talk about it, you think about whether you're both ready for sex, you are safe and responsible about planning for birth control and protecting yourself from STDs. You think you are both ready for sex. Then, you have the first hint of sexual touch and suddenly you freeze. You're scared, you have second thoughts, you want to stop right then and there. Or maybe the opposite happens: you made an agreement to NOT have sex, to practice sexual abstinence and in the heat of the moment, you change your mind and you want to throw off your abstinence ring and break your vows forever. What do you do? You can ignore your feelings, you can ignore you values, you can betray your sexual self, or you can stop and start from the beginning: with sexual communication about who you are at the moment. In the moment of sexual fear, the moment of sexual passion, the moment you change who you are into someone you didn't know that you'd become: you have to be true to your sexual self.

The truth will set you free, sexually speaking.

Speaking up about what you experience, and who you become when you explore your sexuality, will set you free from making sexual mistakes that you will regret. Every situation can change you and every new sexual situation becomes a new beginning with new feelings about who you are at that moment in time. There is a saying, "You can't step into the same river twice," because the water moves and changes every day. You can't know how every sexual situation or any experience will make you feel, but you need to use your sexual voice to speak up about who you are and what you want at the time. Sexual communication is not a one time event, it is an ongoing expression of who you are at any given moment in time. Sex begins with sexual communication. Sex becomes a reflection of your true sexual self when every new beginning begins another new beginning of who you are, the first time and every time.

~~~~~~~~~

> Sexual communication defines your sexual
> self in any given moment.

~~~~~~~~~

## seven

# REAL SEX ED:
# THE SEXUAL DICTIONARY

146

## WHAT IS SEX?

Now that you know that you are a sexual being from birth, you'll want to know about how people express their sexual feelings. Being sexual can mean just feeling sexy, thinking sexual thoughts and having fantasies, looking at other people and their bodies and getting turned on, touching your own body in a way that feels good, being attracted to someone else, kissing and hugging, or wanting to share your feelings with another person with sexual touch. This chapter is a "dictionary," so to speak, of sexual behaviors. Included are many kinds of sexual behaviors, as well as slang names for sex and sexual body parts, including some ethnic slang for sex. Your sexuality may include some, or none, of these behaviors, and may occur now or at sometime in the future, depending on how you choose to express your sexuality.

What most people mean by "losing your virginity" is generally accepted to mean having sexual intercourse, where a man's erect penis enters a woman's vagina and moves in and out in a way that can or may be pleasurable to both people. Truthfully, a lot of teenagers and young people are "virgins" who have nevertheless had a lot of sexual experiences, but they have not had sexual intercourse and so their virginity is technically intact. Some guys and girls enjoy sex by themselves, through masturbation. Many girls and guys enjoy having intimate physical experiences, including kissing and hugging, or they enjoy simply sharing their loving feelings without having any sexual contact. Other teens express their loving feelings through kissing, touching, and sexual touching without having actual sexual intercourse. Really, how people express their sexuality is very personal, very private, and it is only limited by the human imagination. This chapter will discuss the many different ways to express sexuality so that you can start to find the right way for you to express your sexuality in a manner that is appropriate for you.

147

## SEXUAL PARTS

Most children are told: "A man has a penis and a woman has a vagina." A major pet peeve of mine is that most people refer to a woman's sexual parts as her "vagina." A vagina is an "invagination" of skin, or a pocket of skin, inside of your body. A woman doesn't just have a "vagina," which is literally translated as "hole." This is not nearly the entirety of a woman's sexual parts. A woman's outside genitals, in full, are called her "vulva." The vulva is the whole outside area of a woman's genitals including: the clitoris, the clitoral hood (the skin over the clitoris), the urethra (or hole you urinate from), the labia minora or inner "lips," and the labia majora or outer "lips" outside of the vagina. Inside of the labia minora is the vagina, which is only one part of a woman's sexual anatomy. Without the clitoris (or clit in slang terminology), most women don't usually experience ORGASM! So, just referring to woman's genitals as her "vagina" excludes major parts of a woman's sexual body.

I had a horrible yeast infection once and went to a doctor for an exam. My visit to the doctor was triggered by the serious itching and burning I felt when I urinated. After the exam, the male doctor confirmed that I did indeed have a yeast infection and he gave me a prescription and some cream. He told me to rub the cream on my "vagina" to stop the itching. I took the medicine, but I was angry. My red, burning, itching skin was not in my vagina . . . it was on my vulva, which is again outside of my vagina, between the folds of the lips of my labia, and around my urethra and clitoris. OUCH! If I had put it in my vagina, I would have still been burning and suffering. At least I knew to rub the cream on my vulva, on the outside of my genitals, to relieve my pain. I thought, GEEZ . . . he's a doctor . . . at least he should be using the correct words for sexual parts! He just lumped all my parts into one category, like many people: "your vagina."

Recently, I read an article on a new type of plastic surgery, called "female genitalia alteration." This type of plastic surgery is increasing at a greater rate than any other plastic surgery. Basically, it is for women who don't think their genitals look right! They think their labia, or inner or outer lips of their vulva, are too small or too large. Sometimes women think their clitoris or the skin over it, in particular, is too large or too small. This type of surgery alarms and astounds me! As if there is some perfect way for a girl's vulva to look and any other version looks ugly!

In a book written by Betty Dodson, called *Sex for One*, there are several pictures of different types of female vulvas! Betty reveals in her book that, when she was as old as 35, she did not like oral sex, mostly because she was uncomfortable with the appearance of her genitals. She didn't want anyone to look at them: she thought her genitals were deformed because one inner lip was shorter than the other one. She had an ugly image of her genitals, and thus she was embarrassed at the sight of her genitals. She also thought of oral sex as being unsanitary. Fortunately, she had a very sensitive lover who told her that her genitals were "normal" and beautiful. In fact, he showed her several explicit pictures of women with their vulvas displayed. Betty found out that there were several other women who had genitals that look just like hers! She was very relieved to find out she wasn't deformed or ugly. She learned to accept and love the sight and shape and sensations of her vulva.

## SELF EXAMINATION

When I think of women today paying money and getting surgery to change the appearance of their genitals, I find this concept ghastly! Also, when I think of women rejecting the sight of their genitals or being afraid or embarrassed about the sight of their genitals, it is very sad to me. This is why girls need to examine themselves and to know themselves through self-examination and self-exploration. You need to know yourself, your sexual parts, your sexual sensations, and your sexual likes and dislikes. Girls need to get to know their own feelings, to find out how they feel and what they like because someday they might want to share their feelings with a sexual partner.

So girls, get in front of a mirror and look at what you've got! Look at your parts and identify each of them. Look at your vulva and vagina and touch each part to see how it feels. See yourself as you really are and say to yourself that you are beautiful. Tell yourself that you are perfectly made, that you are blessed with physical parts and physical sensations that are God-given and natural. Do not reject yourself and your sexuality.

*Words for Vagina*

- Va-Va
- Cunt
- Hole
- Box

*Words for Vulva*

- Beaver
- Twat

- Pussy
- Snatch

## Words for Breasts

- Tits or titties
- Boobs
- Hooters
- Knockers
- Jugs
- Headlights (refers to erect nipples showing)
- Ta-tas
- Tacos

## Words for Penis

- Dick
- Cock
- Dong
- Schlong
- Wee-Wee
- Willy
- Rod
- Wang
- Wiener
- Peter
- Pecker
- Johnson

## Words for Testicles

- Balls
- Nuts

- Jewels
- Rocks
- Nuggies

## TYPES OF SEXUAL BEHAVIORS

### Fantasies

Fantasies are one of the first ways that people express their sexuality. Fantasies are your thoughts about sex. One of the great things about fantasies is that they are safe: you can't get pregnant, you can't get hurt, you can't get STDs, and you don't have to have anyone's permission to enjoy them! Thinking about sex, and thinking about yourself and other people in a sexual way is a normal part of being a sexual person. Fantasies may be a way for you to explore how you might feel about a person, place or sexual situation. You don't have to act on your fantasies, but you can explore your feelings about sex in your own imagination.

Sometimes fantasies may be just thinking about someone you have a huge crush on. You might think about this person talking to you, and you might rehearse in your mind how you would act. Sometimes fantasies are about someone you know you'll never meet or hook up with, like a movie star, or perhaps the captain of the football team if he moves in social circles you don't care to join. Some fantasies involve a certain place you imagine being romantic or sexy, such as the beach or a mountain cabin. Fantasies can be a fun way to get turned on.

Sometimes fantasies can contain violence or kinky sex. For example, you might fantasize about being tied up in leather and whipped or even raped, or doing that to someone else. Fantasizing about something doesn't mean you really want to act it out. The fantasy may be really exciting, but the fact that this act turns you on doesn't mean you are sick. Many women fantasize about having

151

sex forced on them, but in reality, no one ever wants this to happen. Being raped is very, very different than fantasizing about it. Sometimes a rape fantasy is a way for you to imagine having sex, when in reality, you would never give yourself permission to have sex because you aren't ready or you would have religious guilt.

Almost always, fantasies are a harmless way to explore your feelings about sex and to get sexually excited. It doesn't mean that you're not turned on by your sexual partner or that they're not turned on by you, either. On the other hand, if either one of you only gets turned on by fantasies, then you might have a problem. Fantasies can become a problem if you can't get sexually excited without thinking about them or you are obsessing about certain things that are very disgusting to you and you can't get them off your mind. If you find yourself being stuck on a fantasy that bothers you and you can't seem to have other sexual feelings that are right for you, you should consider talking to a sexuality professional, such as a sex counselor.

## Wet Dreams

Girls and guys, after puberty, have orgasms in their dreams, while they are sleeping. Wow! What a great thing! It's like a freebie in your sleep. Maybe you're having an erotic dream about the guy or gal next to you in science class, and the next thing you know, you are half awake, feeling warm inside, wet outside, and breathing deeply. Isn't this is an awesome thing? Without the hassle of relationships, privacy, masturbation, or anything, your body gets sexually aroused, sometimes just biologically or sometimes through a dream, and gets you off with an orgasm!

Many people think that just guys have "wet dreams," or as they are technically called, "nocturnal emissions." Almost all of the writings about wet dreams are about guys who "come" or ejaculate in their sleep. Wet dreams just sort of start happening to guys when they go through puberty. They will just wake up in the morning and have stickiness and wetness on their penis from the fluid of ejaculation. According to the good old sex researchers, almost all guys will have this happen on a regular basis, and it is "normal."

As a sex researcher and therapist, I have seen very little research or documentation about girls' wet dreams. I am happy to tell you, however, that it does seem to happen to women more and more as they grow older. Maybe this is because women become more sexually enlightened or have a stronger sex drive as they get older, or maybe these wet dreams are simply because they don't have a sexual partner when they are used to having one. The good news is that girls have wet dreams, too.

Wet dreams are a sexual release in the middle of the night. So if a guy says he has "blue balls," meaning he is sexually aroused but did not ejaculate and he is afraid that his balls (or testicles) are going to hurt later, simply tell him not to worry: his body will take care of him tonight and give him a sexual release before he "busts his balls."

## Sex for One

Betty Dodson is the "queen of masturbation" to me. She wrote about masturbation over and over again in the 70s when some of your parents (or grandparents) were first having sexual experiences. Masturbation was a very controversial topic in the 70's, especially since it was widely considered sinful. Besides being against God, masturbation had all sorts of urban myths surrounding it, like if you did it you would go blind or start to permanently drool. Many, many centuries ago, it was thought that sperm contained very, very tiny people inside of it. So, of course, it was sinful to "spill the seed" of the semen, as the Bible says, as that was considered "MURDER." Of course, murder is against one of the Ten Commandments, so masturbation was considered sinful.

Now let's jump into the 21st Century, where we know that

sperm is simply a billion (or so) seeds to be planted, completely un-connected to human life until one penetrates the egg in a woman's womb at the right time and place. Alone, in the middle of a bunch of Kleenex (or a sock), the billions of sperm are as potent as the yellow pollen of spring that unsuccessfully lands on our cars instead of on the fertile and open petals of another flower. No murder. No sin. No blindness. No drooling. These are just dead cells that would die no matter where ejaculation occurred, if outside of a woman. Remember, even when a woman gets pregnant, except in the case of fraternal twins, only one of billions of sperm fertilizes an egg and the rest all die.

As Betty Dodson says, "Masturbation has come of age." She in-troduces her book with: "Masturbation is a primary form of sexual expression. It's not just for kids or those in between lovers or for old people who end up alone. Masturbation is the ongoing love affair that each of us has with ourselves throughout our lifetime" (pg. 3).

Masturbation is having sex with yourself, or touching yourself in a sexual way alone or with a lover present. How you touch yourself in a sexual way is completely up to you and what you want to try and/or explore. Most women use their hands for sexual exploration, to feel their breasts, to feel the sensations of their nipples, to touch the rest of their bodies, and then to continue to genital self-explo-ration. Some women use vibrators or water from a shower massage or bathtub spout for sexual excitement. For a woman, this gener-ally involves stimulation of her clitoris, and it may involve vaginal penetration with her own hand or a dildo. A dildo is a sex toy that looks like a penis. More women have orgasms from clitoral stimula-tion than with penetration into their vaginas, and we'll talk about the different kinds of orgasms for women later in this chapter. But for now, remember that many women bring themselves to orgasm without penetration but only with stimulation to the outside por-tions of their genitals.

For some women, "masturbation" is a negative word. So, there are other words you might want to use for masturbation.

## Words for Female Masturbation

- Self loving
- Self stimulation
- Self pleasuring
- Paddling the pink canoe
- Rubbing off
- Combing the clit
- Vibrating off
- Self touching

## Words for Male Masturbation

- Jacking off
- Jerking Off
- Spanking the monkey
- Choking the chicken
- Bopping the bologna
- Beat the meat
- Flog the hog
- Relieving yourself
- Yanking the plank
- Beating off
- Getting off
- Masturbation
- Self stimulation
- Bobbing the dolphin
- Shining the knob
- Rubbin' the nubbin
- Pounding the mound

Do you notice the big difference in the vocabulary available for guys and girls for sexual parts, and especially masturbation? I took a linguistics class about 20 years ago in college. It was about how language was developed and used in different cultures. I never thought I would ever be able to use any of the knowledge from that class (do you know what I mean?) which was required for college graduation, but what I learned is that when cultures have many words for one thing, that one thing is important and significant in their culture. For example, in most of America, we have one word for snow: snow. Eskimos, apparently, have many words for snow, because it is such an important part of their life and culture. Since men have so many more phrases for masturbation, it's obvious that male masturbation is seen as more important and acceptable in our culture for men. Women need to make masturbation more IMPORTANT AND SIGNIFICANT for themselves. After all, we have much superior abilities to have more orgasms than guys anyway (which is described below)!

When it comes to masturbation, first, you have to start with permission. While some religions preach that masturbation is a sin, science has destroyed the myth that masturbation is physically bad for you. In fact, it is essential to your sexual health to KNOW yourself and KNOW what you like and what you don't like. Even some religions will allow masturbation, if it is considered useful for the preservation of a marriage. Most importantly . . . it is essential to stop being EMBARRASSED about "touching yourself." You will notice that NO GUYS are embarrassed about this (unless they are caught right in the act, like in the movie *American Pie*). As a young woman, you may need to work on developing a healthy attitude toward self touch, and to develop your own vocabulary and phrases to claim its importance in your life.

~~~~~~~~~~~

> As women, we need to love our genitals and sex . . .
> and to demand love and respect for our sexual parts
> from others.

~~~~~~~~~~~

*Words or Phrases People Use for Sex*

- Making love
- Sexual intercourse
- Having sex
- Sleeping together
- Fucking
- Sexing
- Screwing
- Banging
- Shagging
- Boning
- Jumping your bones
- Let me hit it
- Tapping some of that
- Doing the nasty
- Humping
- Getting a piece of ass
- Getting some
- Doing it
- Chopping-"Hey, you wanna chop?"
- Cuttin'/cutting-"Can I cut?"
- Slamming-"Can I slam?"
- Hittin it/hit it-"Can I hit that?"
- Beatin/beating

## ORAL SEX

When my daughter was 12 years old, she asked me, "Are blow jobs bad?" As a parent, I was a little surprised by this question, especially from a girl in 7th grade, but I thought it was an excellent inquiry. She told me that guys at school would often say "Blow me!" to someone they wanted to insult or didn't like. She had also heard of older girls giving guys blowjobs in the bathrooms at the high school football games. Naturally, being raised by a pack of sex therapists (her stepfather and a few of our friends are sex therapists too), she felt comfortable in asking my opinion.

My answer was, "It depends." Of course, I explained to her that "blow job" was the slang term for oral sex performed on a man. Specifically, I explained that a blow job was rubbing up and down on a guy's penis with your hand and mouth, sometimes while fondling the guy's testicles, usually until he reached orgasm, at which time he would ejaculate. Certainly, she'd already gotten the whole sex talk by the time she was 12, so she knew all about the need to be ready for a sexual relationship before engaging in one. It was explained to her that oral sex IS sex, which is an intimate physical expression of your feelings toward someone in a private and personal way. So I explained that all the things that are important regarding readiness and decisions for sex have to be considered when sharing oral sex, too. The only major difference is that you can't get pregnant from giving/having oral sex, or "giving blow jobs."

Besides the emotional and relationship considerations in oral sex, which are discussed fully in Chapter 4, there are the physical considerations of oral sex. Since oral sex, or giving blowjobs, includes the ejaculation of seminal fluid or come, oral sex is not safe sex. You can get sexually transmitted diseases from oral sex. Many girls do not realize that giving a blowjob is physically dangerous and that you can get STDs, including AIDS, from oral sex. This aspect of risk does make blowjobs "bad." Now, girls have a choice in oral sex, of whether to stop performing oral sex when a guy is about ready to ejaculate or to take the ejaculate into her mouth, and then she can decide whether to swallow it or spit it out. That is a personal choice. Guys prefer it when a girl allows them to ejaculate while their penis is still inside of her mouth. Part of this is the continuity of sexual excitement, and part of it is because it makes a guy feel more "accepted" by a girl, and part of it might just be the taboo of coming into an orifice that our culture has traditionally not designated for such behavior. No matter what you do, the "pre-ejaculate" or fluid that seeps out of a penis when a guy is excited can transmit STDs. For that reason, a condom should always be used for oral sex as well as vaginal sex. There are flavored condoms, such as chocolate or watermelon that are made for this purpose.

So, to repeat my daughter's question, are blow jobs "bad?" Yes, if you are being irresponsible and practicing unsafe sex or you are not ready for a sexual relationship. Any type of sexual contact may be bad if you are not ready for it. Some people are grossed out by this sex act and some people love it. Some religions frown upon or forbid oral sex altogether, so it is important that you understand your religion's values regarding oral sex and heed your own religious morals.

Are blow jobs "bad?" No, oral sex can be an intimate expression of love and pleasuring each other for a couple ready for a sexual relationship. Yet, for some reason, some girls and guys view giving blowjobs as not really having sex. It is SEX, and it carries all of the physical and emotional consequences of sex. Sometimes, girls who do everything but have sexual intercourse, especially by giving guys blowjobs, hold themselves out to be superior to others by virtue of having an intact hymen (that is, a girl is technically a virgin until her hymen is broken or torn). A nickname for these girls is "virgin whores." So, you need to keep in mind that this harsh name indicates that, although you might not consider oral sex real sex, others do and will hold you accountable and talk about you as if you were sexually active.

### Words or Phrases for Oral Sex on a Girl

- Cunnilingus
- Oral sex
- Eating pussy
- Eating her out
- Going down on her
- Muff diving
- Eating at the "Y"

### Words or Phrases for Oral Sex on a Guy

- Fellatio
- Oral sex
- Blowjob
- BJ
- Sucking him off
- Giving "head"

### Words or Phrases for Casual Sex

Casual sex is a term used when people have sex outside a committed relationship, such as marriage, engagement, or a monogamous relationship. A monogamous relationship means that two people are committed to each other and have no other sexual partners. Whether or not you have such a sexual arrangement will depend on your own moral associations with uncommitted sex and your comfort level with such behavior. I have told you that sex within a caring relationship contributes to the experience, but the truth is that many people have sex outside of relationships in order to have sexual closeness without the responsibilities that accompany a deeper relationship. You will have to consider these things for yourself relative to your own conditions for sex:

- Friends with Benefits
- Sportssexing
- Bed Buddies
- Sportsfucking
- Fuckbuddies
- Playing the field

## SEXUAL RESPONSE AND ORGASMS

Girls experience a lot of different sexual responses and orgasms. As stated previously, our bodies are wired for sex, and as you get more and more excited, or aroused, and then finish the sexual act and release sexual tension, your body will go through a series of physical responses to sex, called the sexual response cycle (Masters and Johnson, 1966). There are four basic stages of sexual response: 1. Sexual desire, 2. Sexual arousal, 3. Orgasms, 4. Relaxation. Each person is different and every situation is different, and you will not go through the whole cycle of responses every time you feel excited. Sometimes you might have a lot of excitement but not really get physically aroused or even come close to having an orgasm. At another time, you might not even feel so excited but an orgasm just seems to happen. The sexual response cycle is a process that each person experiences uniquely, but it is important to understand and learn what may happen when you get sexually excited in order to be prepared for sexual situations and your body's response to them. Most girls know what it feels like to get sexually excited, but sexual responses range from feeling sexual desire to feeling physically turned on to having an orgasm or climax; and you need to be prepared for what happens to a woman's body in each stage.

161

## Sexual Desire

The first stage of sexual response is sexual desire. Sometimes you might be thinking about something sexy or looking at someone who turns you on, and you may feel sexual excitement or desire as a result. Your "conditions" for sex usually need to be met (see Chapter 4). Desire is the feeling of wanting sexual touch, by yourself or with a partner, and sometimes it is called being horny. When a girl is horny, sometimes she just wants to be close to someone and to be kissed and hugged, or she may have stronger feelings and desire sexual contact. Sexual desire can be something that happens several times a week or not at all, depending on what is going on in your life at that time or what you are doing and with whom. When you are not with your partner, you may feel a sense of longing to be with them or to talk to them. Sometimes, desire is a mild feeling until you start to fantasize about sex, or until you get into kissing or hugging or having sexual touch, by yourself or with someone else, and you want to be emotionally and physically close to another person.

Stronger sexual desire can be a physical feeling of pulsating, throbbing or aching coming from your clitoris or vagina. When you get into big time making out, sexual desire can lead you to want more physical touch or to try sex, even before you get a chance to think about what you want to do emotionally or rationally. So, you need to remember this is a normal response to physical touching, and you need to think about how far you want to go in a sexual situation before you are really turned on. You need to think about your response before you put yourself in the position to respond, or you may make a choice merely because your body is responding to lots of physical stimulus rather than because you are doing what is right for you. This is a very important difference in men and women. A lot of women don't get horny or a feeling of desire, until after they begin to make-out, kiss, or get sexually aroused. Girls and women often need a transition from thinking about everyday life to thinking about sex. Usually having emotional intimacy, then physical touch helps girls have a transition and feel sexual desire. On the other side of the sexual desire differences, some girls do think about sex a lot, and have strong sexual desires. Some girls have strong physical sexual urges, and they might be more sexually aggressive. In other cases, girls may be aggressive with guys to manipulate them with sex, to get what they want: emotional closeness.

## Sexual Arousal

Sexual arousal means feeling sensations of physical excitement or being "turned on." Physical sexual arousal shows for guys when they get an erection. For girls, sexual excitement shows when their vagina gets lubricated or "wet." When girls get aroused, their vaginas get moist and their vaginas expand: the vaginal walls get thicker and expand in length, making the penetration of a finger or penis possible. Usually, if you are attracted to someone, you will begin to get sexually aroused just from talking and being with each other. Most girls will get physically aroused with touch that doesn't include sexual areas, including kissing, hugging, and caressing of the face, hair, arms, legs and body. Sometimes physical arousal happens from visual stimulation or looking at your partner's body. Physical arousal also usually happens with touching of the sexual areas: the breasts, buttocks, clitoris, vulva, or vagina. Sometimes girls can feel when they get aroused, but a lot of girls don't know if they're "wet" unless their underwear is wet or they feel themselves with their fingers.

163

> For some girls, they do not feel sexual desire or the wanting of sex, until after they feel sexual and physical excitement.

*Sources of Sexual Arousal*

- Touch
- Smell
- Sight
- Sound
- Kissing
- Music
- Sexy movies
- A deep emotional connection
- Sexual fantasies

Some girls are not able to have physical sexual arousal. That is, they do not feel excited, they don't get wet or lubricated, and they are unable to have an orgasm. A number of factors may cause a lack of sexual excitement, but a lack of arousal usually means a girl is not ready or prepared for vaginal penetration, emotionally or physically. The most common reasons are:

- Too nervous to get relaxed and aroused
- Conflicts with sexual values
- Difficult past sexual experiences
- Simply not ready for sexual touch
- A lack of emotional feelings that lead to sexual excitement
- Your mind says yes, but body says no
- Physical problem with lubrication (uncommon in young women).

## Orgasms

The next stage of sexual response is the orgasm. Generally, it is accepted that there are two different types of orgasms: clitoral and vaginal. A clitoral orgasm is a peak of sexual arousal that usually happens following touching, rubbing or stimulation of the clitoris. The second type of orgasm is a vaginal orgasm, which results from penetration and stimulation inside of the vagina with a penis or a finger or a dildo. Women can also have orgasms from anal sex. Defining an "orgasm" is very difficult, as it is experienced very differently among women. Physically, an orgasm is a peak of sexual excitement and muscle tension, with a series of muscle contractions, including the contraction of the muscles in your uterus, though the vagina, clitoris and pelvic regions, and a release of those muscles. Some women report feeling like fireworks went off and explosions shot through their bodies. Other women report feeling their muscles tense and release and that the experience was "OK." However, orgasm usually feels very good, and it can be very intense. If it is just OK . . . you might need more practice or experience, with yourself or a partner.

165

Girls may have orgasms from very young ages, as early as 3 or 4, but most women do not report experiencing orgasms until after puberty. Not all women have orgasms. Approximately 78% of women under 30 have clitoral orgasms, but with instruction, practice and sometimes the use of a vibrator almost all women can have clitoral orgasms. Fewer women experience vaginal orgasms than clitoral orgasms. About 30% of women have them all the time, 30% of women have them some of the time, and the rest of women don't experience the sensation at all. Again, with practice and guidance, many women can have vaginal orgasms, too. Some women must have stimulation of the clitoris, through body or hand rubbing during intercourse, so that they can have an orgasm with vaginal penetration, but the orgasm comes from clitoral stimulation.

Some women have orgasms only by themselves and not with a partner, that is, they may have orgasms through masturbation, but not with a sexual partner. Many women do not have orgasms all the time, with every sexual experience. Sadly, most teenage girls do not have orgasms with their male partners. Usually, this is from a lack of experience, girls not knowing how to have an orgasm and boys not knowing how to give them one. This situation is a result of girls not knowing their own bodies or of girls not using their sexual voice to tell their partners what they want. And this is also a result of guys not knowing or caring about what they are doing as regards a girl's needs. Girls, this needs to change, and YOU need to be the ones to change it. Remember: if you're not getting anything out of sex, this is called bad sex!

It is really not decided in sex research circles why some women have vaginal orgasms and others don't. Many researchers believe that women have a "G-spot," or Grafenberg Spot, which is a place about 2 inches inside of the vagina on the belly button side that causes intense vaginal orgasms when it is stimulated by a finger or penis. Some women have orgasms without any physical touch at all. They can "think off." They can have an orgasm simply through sexual fantasy. Some women have orgasms without genital touch, such as via the touching of their nipples. Many women have the ability to have more than one orgasm, or multiple orgasms. When I was much younger, I thought multiple orgasms meant you had more than one at a time. I couldn't understand how women did that and I felt somewhat inferior that I could only have one at a time. Later, I realized multiple orgasms meant having one after another: maybe one, maybe two, maybe even 15 orgasms in one day. Women are different than men in this way, in that they can physically have as many orgasms as they would like to have in one sexual encounter. Men are usually pretty much done after one or at most a few ejaculations. They simply run out of semen after awhile and have to wait for it to be replenished.

## FEMALE EJACULATION

Some women ejaculate fluid from the urethra (where urine comes out) during orgasm. Some researchers have found that this occurs when the G-spot is stimulated. This fluid has been found not to be urine but a fluid unique to intense sexual pleasuring. It is normal, just like a man's ejaculation during intercourse is normal.

# MORE SEXUAL WORDS

**Abstinence:** Not engaging in sexual relations, especially sexual intercourse. "Continuous" abstinence means not ever having sex. 'Periodic' abstinence means not having sexual intercourse during some periods of time, which is not safe sex.

**Anal sex:** Stimulation or penetration of the anus

**AIDS:** Acquired Immune Deficiency Syndrome, a sexually transmitted disease that causes death.

**Bisexuality:** Having sexual relationships with both sexes

**Blow jobs:** Oral sex. Oral sex on a guy is sucking or licking his penis. Oral sex on a girl is kissing and licking her clitoris.

**Clitoris (KLIT-o-ris):** A small, very sensitive piece of skin located at the top of the vulva, just below the pubic bone. It is more easily found with touch, rather than sight because it is small, but very sensitive to touch, often tingling on contact. The sole purpose of the clitoris is for sexual arousal, and it is very important for sexual pleasure.

**Condom:** A rubber, latex, or animal skin sheath made to cover the penis and prevent pregnancy and reduce the risk of sexually transmitted diseases

**Dildo:** A sexual "toy" that is generally made out of plastic or soft or hard rubber that is in the shape of a penis. It is for use in vaginal or anal penetration during sex.

**Diaphragm:** Birth control device, shaped like a small dome, made out of latex to fit inside the vagina and over the cervix.

**Erection:** When a guy's penis is hard and stiff

**Ejaculation:** When semen comes out of the urinary opening (or small hole) on the head of the penis.

**Foreplay:** Any physical touching, including sexual touching, that does not include sexual intercourse.

**HIV:** Human acquired immunodeficiency virus. This is the virus that many scientists believe causes AIDS. When someone "gets AIDS," they first get the HIV virus. Many people live with HIV for several years before it "turns into" AIDS.

**Hymen:** A membrane, or layer of skin, that partially covers the inside of the vagina. The hymen is generally opened when a girl loses her virginity, but it can be opened through vigorous athletic activity or tampon use. Slang: "cherry" or "maidenhead."

**Monogamy:** Both sexual partners having sex with only each other; not having other sexual partners.

**Outercourse:** A newer term referring to sexual play that does not involve anal or vaginal intercourse.

**Semen:** Semen is the fluid ejaculated when a male has an orgasm.

**STDs:** Sexually transmitted diseases (See Chapter 8). Also called "STIs," for sexually transmitted infections, which is the more current, politically correct term.

**Transgendered:** A person who feels they were born in the wrong body. For girls, it means they have female genitalia, but inside they feel like a boy. Also called transexuals or "trannies" for slang.

**Vibrator:** A "sexual toy" that may be in the shape of a dildo, except that is has batteries and vibrates. Or a wand shaped device that vibrates, usually used for clitoral stimulation: may be plugged in or powered by batteries.

**Virgin Sex:** Sex for the first time. Virgin sex can be any sexual experience, including self-touch, mutual sexual touching, oral sex, and sexual intercourse. Some people think "real sex" is considered sex that involves sexual intercourse, but the truth is that all sexual acts are a form of sexual behavior and thus virgin sex is the first time you do any of these things. However, you only lose your virginity, technically speaking, when you have intercourse for the first time.

## *eight*

# STDS, SAFER SEX, AND BIRTH CONTROL

**V**irgin sex, no regrets, is up to <u>YOU</u>.

- **Y**our sexual voice needs to be loud and clear in both giving permission for sex and insisting on using protection when YOU are ready for sex.
- **O**nly you can decide when you are emotionally and physically ready for sex and to be responsible with sex.
- **U**se protection against STDs and pregnancy each and every time you have sex.

First, your sexual voice is essential, to protect yourself emotionally and physically with sex. Speak up, say what you want and don't want, to give permission for sex or to say no and wait. Always speak up and insist that you use protection against STDs and pregnancy. Second, only you can decide to be responsible to practice safer sex, physically. No one else is going to be as concerned with your safety, as you. Third, make it a choice to use protection from STDs and pregnancy each and every time you have sexual interaction. Not regretting sex demands your taking responsibility for being safe and healthy sexually.

~~~~~~~~~~~~~~~~~~~~~~~~

> Remember: 90% of girls who are sexually active and do not use birth control will become pregnant within one year. 25% of girls contract a sexually transmitted disease as a teenager.

~~~~~~~~~~~~~~~~~~~~~~~~

## SEXUALLY TRANSMITTED DISEASES (STDS)

STDs and sex are like handling a gun: always assume a gun is loaded when handling it. Always assume your sexual partner has an STD, unless they have been very recently tested, and tested negatively for having an STD. Every sexual partner is only as healthy as their most recent sexual encounter. Every sexual encounter exposes an individual to every previous sexual encounter of their partner. Everybody is vulnerable to STDs unless they protect themselves from infections, each and every time they have sex.

STDs affect all women, especially young women, but they also affect minorities disproportionately, and consistently more frequently. Black women have significantly higher rates of sexually transmitted diseases than white or non-white Hispanic women. Black women are the fastest growing group of women to be infected with HIV, who are 7 times more likely to contract HIV than white women. Black women are also more likely to contract gonorrhea (18x more likely), chylamdia (5x more likely), and syphilis (Nakashima, Rolfs, Flock, et al, 1996; alanguttmacher.com, 2006). All girls need to protect themselves against STDs, but girls of color need to be aware that they are especially vulnerable to sexually transmitted infections.

## STDs—Jake's Story

Jake was 12 years old when he was influenced by, as he says, the glamorizing of drugs and sex and became rebellious. This led him to experimenting with drugs and sex. Jake's parents had divorced when he was 3. His mother was a struggling, working woman who tried her best to support her three kids, but the family was poor. Theirs was a poverty-stricken household with not much to do for excitement, so Jake was attracted to sex and drugs to try to be cool and fit in. Jake was brought in by the wrong crowd and was introduced to sex by a 15 year-old girl. "Kara" had been having sexual intercourse for a couple of years, which made her very experienced by the time she met Jake. After Kara coaxed him into having sex with her, Jake felt that he had been taken advantage of, and to make things worse, their sexual experience resulted in a STD scare for him. There was a group orgy at a party, where everyone was drunk or high, and several of the kids involved were discovered to have an STD. The rumor was that Kara had AIDS and had spread it to several sexual partners.

Jake realized he was going to have to get tested for a sexually transmitted disease, particularly AIDS. Jake's middle school counselor told him where the health department and clinic were located and he went there by himself on his bicycle. It was traumatic for this 12 year-old boy to have to go to the local free health clinic for a STD examination. Jake's family didn't have the money to go to a private doctor, and he had to sit in a huge public waiting room for two hours, where lots of other people were also waiting to see the free doctor. During the STD examination, Jake had to have blood samples taken, his penis was examined for any sores or blisters, and his anus was looked at and prodded with the doctor's finger. Jake was also asked about the circumstances surrounding his potential contraction of an STD.

The whole examination was extremely embarrassing, as well

as scary because Jake was thinking he might have a STD the entire time. The biggest deal was that Jake had to tell his mother that he had sexual intercourse, about Kara, and about the party where everyone was having sex. Telling his mom was the most traumatic part of everything. Jake thought about running away to avoid having to tell her what he did, but he was more afraid of dying from AIDS or something else if he didn't tell her and get her help. As it turned out, one of Jake's friends, "Nick," had called his mother earlier that day. Nick had called her from the clinic because he was there to get tested too (Nick had been at the party as well). So, Jake's mother had already gotten the news and was over the initial shock when Jake talked to her. Fortunately, Jake did not get an STD, but the situation could have turned out differently. After that, Jake stayed away from sex for a long time.

Obviously, one of the worst negative consequences of sex can be acquiring a sexually transmitted disease since you can die from some of them. Sexually transmitted diseases are diseases that are passed from person to person through sexual contact, and specifically, from the exchange of sexual bodily fluids. Sexually transmitted diseases are called "STDs," "VD" for venereal disease, and "STIs" for sexually transmitted infections. Another common slang for STDs is called "getting burned." This book will provide just a brief overview of STDs for you, since there are lots of other resources on STDs and this is not the major focus of this book. The Internet has many health sites that offer more extensive information on STDs, and you can also find information about STDs at the public library.

Whether you are having sex for the first time or you've had many sexual partners, you want to protect yourself from STDs. STDs can kill you, make you infertile, or maybe just make your crotch itch like crazy and burn when you urinate! Some STDs can make you sterile for life, meaning you can't have children! A lot of times, you can't tell if you have an STD or when someone else has one just by looking at them. Some STDs that are immediately infectious but remain undetectable (you don't know you have it), such as HIV or syphilis, can be transmitted or given to sexual partners without your knowledge. That's why STDs spread so fast.

Once someone is infected with an STD, they can give it to their sexual partner. STDs are spread through close skin-to-skin genital contact or by bodily fluids shared during vaginal, oral and anal sex, which include blood, semen, and vaginal fluids. Every time you have sex with someone, when it comes to STDs, biologically speaking, both of you are having sex with every previous sexual partner you have ever had, every previous sexual partner your sexual partners have had, every previous sexual partner their previous sexual partners have ever had, and so on. Since there is no way that you can know about everyone's sexual history and sexual health, you need to take care of your own health and protect the future health of those people you care about or love by practicing safe or safer sex. That is why if either of you have engaged in sexually risky behavior, it is best to be tested for STDs to avoid spreading diseases. It is very important to go to a doctor or even a free clinic to have a medical screening for STDs. Having an STD can have an effect on your whole life, including your health, your future sexual relationships, and your ability to have children.

Even if it doesn't seem that important at the moment, being irresponsible now with unsafe sexual practices can affect you for your entire life.

# COMMON TYPES OF SEXUALLY TRANSMITTED DISEASES

## HIV/AIDS

HIV and AIDS is the most feared STD, because there is no cure. Although people are living longer and better quality lives while living with AIDS, medical treatment is expensive, requiring an extensive routine of many drugs, if you can afford them, and, ultimately, they may not work. Human immunodeficiency virus, also called HIV, is a virus that destroys your immune system. Without an immune system, which protects you from illnesses and diseases, your body can get very sick from ordinary infections, or rare types of infections. People who have HIV can become very ill to the point that they can't fight disease. When the body is very ill from HIV and doesn't have enough healthy cells to fight germs, HIV turns into acquired immune deficiency syndrome or AIDS. People don't actually die from AIDS, they die from having a weak immune system and getting a disease they can't fight off.

You can get HIV in the same way that you get other STDs: through the sharing of bodily fluids during sexual activity. Also, you can get infected with HIV from having contact with the body fluids, including blood, of someone who has HIV, either from sexual activity or through a cut, tear, or other broken skin opening. HIV can also be passed on to a child during pregnancy or from breast milk. Infections from blood usually happen when needles are shared with intravenous drug use, in blood transfusions, and from even tiny amounts of blood shared during sexual activity. People usually get HIV from sexual intercourse of any kind, and sharing infected drug needles. All too often, people are really afraid of being around people who have HIV or AIDS and just getting it from every day contact. HIV isn't like catching a cold: you can't get it from hugging, breathing the same air, sharing a glass, or just hanging out with someone who has it. Michael Basso's book,

*The Underground Guide to Teenage Sexuality*, gives a great and easily understandable explanation on HIV and AIDS.

> HIV can be avoided by not having intercourse or oral sex, not using other people's drug needles, and always using protection if you have any sexual contact that involves exchanging bodily fluids.

Every teen can learn from other teens, and their experiences, to learn to make better choices about sex, especially when it comes to the HIV virus and AIDS. To read more about teens are stories on AIDS, check out the website: http://www.hivaids.webcentral.com.au/text/stories.html. Teens get HIV because they have unprotected sexual contact, including oral sex, anal sex, and sexual intercourse, and they have been reckless sometimes just once, and *they simply thought it wouldn't happen to them.*

## Chlamydia

Chlamydia is the most common bacterial STD, infecting up to one in seven women under 30 years old. Symptoms include itching, burning, painful urination, abdominal pain, or a vaginal discharge that may smell funky. Often people feel no symptoms and they don't know they have it. When it is treated with drugs, it causes no lifelong problems. However, if it is untreated, it can cause a lot of damage to your reproductive system and make you infertile, which means you will never be able to have children. Sexually active teens need to be checked regularly for STDs, especially Chlamydia, since is it so common and it may cause permanent damage.

## Jackie's Story

Jackie was a close friend of mine when I was young, and I knew her when I became pregnant with my first child. I was 25, married, and happily pregnant with my daughter, Katie. Of course, Jackie was very happy and excited for me, too, except for one thing: Jackie couldn't have any children. Jackie got burned and had an STD when she was 20 years old. She didn't realize she had it until she became very sick with painful abdominal cramps and ended up in the emergency room. Jackie found out she had "pelvic inflammatory disease," or PID. PID happens when a sexually transmitted disease, such as a chlamydia infection progresses untreated, causing an infection in the ovaries and fallopian tubes. Jackie was successfully treated with medication, but she was told she might have fertility problems due to the severity of her infection. She found out five years later that she was infertile, and she was unable to have children.

Although I was elated about being pregnant, it was hard for me to be around Jackie, at times, because I knew she was sad about not being able to have a child of her own, because of a mistake she made when she was 19. Jackie later adopted a child, and became a great mother later in her life, but it was still a loss for her that she never had biological children with her husband.

There is no nice way to present this story: it is terrible, it is negative, but it is real. What happened to Jackie is one of the sad realities and potential consequences from sexual behavior. You need to know and understand the seriousness of sexually transmitted diseases and their potential impact on your life.

## Genital Herpes

Herpes is a STD that doesn't go away. Once you have it, you have it for life. There is no cure for herpes, although it is not life threatening. Herpes is a virus, and one out of four adults is infected with it. One kind of herpes is common cold sores on the mouth, also called fever blisters or canker sores. The other kind of herpes is genital herpes, which are painful blisters, sores, or red-rimmed bumps on the penis, vulva, anus, and even the mouth. Most people do not know that genital herpes can be transmitted from oral-genital contact, meaning you can get herpes from someone who has what looks like a cold sore, during oral sex. It is estimated that one third of "cold sores" on the mouth are now actually the genital herpes type. This means that if someone receives oral sex from someone with a "cold sore or fever blister" on their mouth, they can get genital herpes!

Herpes is very contagious, and spreads from skin to skin contact with the blisters or bumps. Because it is so contagious, you must be very careful not to spread the infection to other parts of your body, such as your eyes (you can go blind!), or to other people. Condoms can help to prevent the spread of herpes, but sometimes condoms don't cover the place where the blister or bump occurs on the pelvic area, vulva (or mouth!).

The bad thing about herpes is that it isn't a one shot deal. Once you have it, most people get recurrent outbreaks for life. Typically, a person may have one or two outbreaks per year, when they are under stress or physically run down. Some people never get a second outbreak, but some people have outbreaks every month! Some people have the disease, but never experience any symptoms, although they can spread it to other people without knowing it. The first herpes outbreak is typically the worst, with painful blisters, pelvic soreness, itching, burning, and even flu like symptoms. Subsequent outbreaks may only be red bumps, but with itching or burning. Untreated, the sores last about 10 days, but with medication, sores begin to disappear in 2 to 4 days. Medication can be used every day to control having any outbreaks.

## Genital Warts

Genital warts are caused by a virus called human papilloma virus or HPV. HPV stays in a person's system for life, too, so warts can recur. While there are many different types of warts, genital warts can form and grow on a person's genitals, including the pelvic area, the anus, the vulva, and inside of the vagina. Genital warts are also very contagious and spread through skin to skin contact. Like herpes, they can be spread with oral-genital contact. Genital warts can be big or very small cauliflower-like bumps, that may form in clusters or a bunch all together. The bumps are usually painless, but they can itch. The warts have to be removed by a doctor, which can be very painful, due to the sensitivity in the region. As with herpes, condoms can be used to avoid protection against genital warts, but the condom may give only partial protection.

One of the bad things about HPV is that is has been associated with an increased risk of cervical cancer later in life for women. It has also been associated with cancer of the vulva, and anal cancer. If you have been infected with warts, it is very important to have regular pelvic exams to check for problems throughout your life (Bell, 1998).

HPV is one of the fastest growing STDs, especially among college aged students. Often, people do not even know they have HPV until they are tested for it, as many people do not have any symptoms; they are simply "carriers" of the virus, meaning they have the virus, but they have not had any outbreaks of warts. One research study showed that 33% of college aged girls tested for HPV at a college health center had HPV, and most likely, very few of them knew they had it (alanguttmacher.org, 2006). Fortunately, there is now a new vaccine that protects girls and women against HPV, that I recommend ALL girls be given to protect your future health.

## Trichomanos Vaginitis (TV)

Called "trich" or "trick" by slang, trichomanos vaginitis is among the most common STDs, found in up to 33% of college women screened for the infection. Caused by a tiny parasite found in the vagina or urethra (hole where urine comes out), it is similar to a yeast infection. TV causes itching, burning of the vulva and produces a smelly discharge that can be yellowish-green in color. Other symptoms include redness, pain with urination, and pain with sex, and tenderness in the lower abdomen. One half of women infected with trich have no symptoms, but they are "carriers" and can pass the infections along to others. Men can be carriers and pass it along as well, without even knowing they have it. Untreated, the infection can cause cystitis, painful urination, but there are no long term health effects. Trichomoniasis is easily treated with antibiotics when it is detected.

## Gonorrhea

Gonorrhea is another bacterial infection that is passed through penis-vagina intercourse, anal sex and oral sex. Gonorrhea of the throat is becoming more common with more girls giving guys oral sex and not realizing that STDs are spread from the transmission of bodily fluids, including in the mouth. Oral sex is not safe sex! Symptoms of gonorrhea, also known as the clap or drip, include a funky smelling discharge with pus in it, and painful, burning urination. Many girls do not know they have it, and have no symptoms, and some guys have no symptoms, either. As with chlamydia, serious pelvic infections and scarring of the reproductive organs can occur, causing infertility or an inability to have children. Gonorrhea can be treated with antibiotics, with both partners taking the drugs to get rid of it.

## Hepatitis B

Hepatitis B is a virus that can infect a person's liver, causing a serious illness, and even death. Hepatitis B is spread through sexual practices that exchange bodily fluids, including kissing, all types of intercourse, oral sex, and sharing of blood. Hepatitis is common among interveneous drug users (injecting drugs into veins with a needle), and people who practice anal sex. Most people don't realize they have hepatitis because it is a lot like having the flu. Symptoms include a sick stomach, no appetite, headaches, dizziness, and being tired, but also soreness in your liver area, dark colored urine, and yellowish eyes or skin. Hepatitis B is usually curable, but the medical treatment is very long and extensive, including two to three months of treatment (Bell, 1998). It is highly recommended that young women get vaccinated against Hepatitis B, as it is an easy way to prevent a disease that can have many complications.

## Pubic Lice

Commonly known as "crabs," these are tiny little animals that jump from one body to another, and generally live in hair, including pubic hair and eyelashes. Pubic lice is highly contagious and is spread from close contact with another person who has it. You will know if you have crabs because they itch like crazy! Pubic lice is treatable and curable, with over the counter and prescription drugs. You can ask your pharmacist for help or go to a doctor. It is really important that all of your clothing, bedding, carpeting, stuffed animals or anything cloth be cleaned in hot soapy water or put in tightly sealed plastic bags to totally get rid of all the little bugs and their eggs, which can live for days.

## Syphilis

Another bacterial infection, it is spread by sexual or skin contact from a person who has the rash or sores of the disease. Drugs can completely cure the illness, if it is caught in an early stage. Untreated, syphilis is a very serious, life threatening disease, causing damage to internal organs, including your sexual organs, and causing birth defects. Later, it can also damage the heart, brain, and nervous system, even leading to insanity. Early treatment is very important.

## SAFEST SEX

There is no such thing as totally safe sex with a partner.

If you are engaging in sexual practices, you are taking a risk that you will get a STD or get pregnant. You will also risk that you may be emotionally hurt by sex.

**Abstinence.** The absolute surest way to avoid ever contracting a STDs or having an unwanted pregnancy is to not be sexually active, which is called sexual abstinence, or literally, abstaining from sex. The safest sexual activity is to participate in sexual behaviors that do not allow the transmission of fluids between two partners. The safest sex is where you do not engage in any contact of the genitals, including not kissing the genitals with the mouth. For example, sexual contact with each other's genitals through clothing, by touching or rubbing each other through clothing, is a safe way to express sexual affection. Dry kissing (no tongue), holding, or dancing, as long as sexual fluids are not exchanged and sexual skin does not touch, are safe sexual behaviors. Some people are afraid of getting AIDS from wet kissing, but most doctors believe the quality of the HIV virus in saliva is too low to cause HIV.

Abstinence is only effective as safer sex only if it is practiced *each* and *every* time. Period. It is important to know that many teenagers plan to abstain from sex, and to be safe from sexual risks through sexual abstinence, but for a thousand different reasons, this plan changes. Abstinence is only effective if is it used continuously, or all the time, which, in reality, often does not happen. For that reason, it is important to have a back-up plan, in case you change your mind in a given situation.

**Masturbation.** Having sex with yourself poses no threat of acquiring a sexually transmitted disease. Masturbation in front of your partner, without touching each other or sharing sexual fluids, is also safe sex.

## SAFER SEX PRACTICES

You can be responsible for yourself and you can learn to practice "safer" sex. You can learn what is sexually dangerous or risky and NOT engage in those behaviors. Please remember that sometimes teenagers can be moody or depressed, in part due to hormonal changes, and consequently, at times it seems like it doesn't matter what happens to you or if you hurt yourself from sex. Or you might just want to be with someone on the spur of the moment, without thinking about what could happen. Please never forget, however, that that if you wait 24 hours, you might feel differently about your life or the person you are with right now. Also, even if it doesn't seem like anyone in the world cares about you, you probably do have family and friends who love you and want you to stay healthy and alive. If nothing else, care about yourself: you are here on this Earth for a reason, and while you're a teenager, you probably have very little idea of whom or what you may become.

# Safer Sex Guide

- Start with sexual relations negotiations: discuss STDs, safer sex and sexual practices, the use of condoms, cheating (sex with others outside of the relationship), and birth control with your partner.

- Practice monogamy. Monogamy means two people only have sex with each other. If both of you are absolutely certain neither of you is infected with a STD, and you are certain neither of you has any other partners, which can be very hard to know because of the honesty issue, even when you love each other, then you will both be safe from STDs.

- Use a condom each and every time there is sexual contact of the genitals, including oral and anal sex.

- Identify your own past potentially risky sexual behaviors. If there is any risk, see a doctor or visit a clinic before having unprotected sex.

- Ask your sexual partners about their potential risk of disease. If there is any risk, have your partner visit a clinic or see a doctor for STD testing before you consent to have sex with them.

- Limit your sexual partners. The more sexual partners you have, the greater your chance for STDs. Also for this reason, avoid partners who have had multiple partners.

- Postpone any exchange of bodily fluids until lab tests verify that you are both free of STDs. HIV testing, for example, is a two step process, and you have to wait six months for your second HIV test to be reasonably certain that you do not have the virus.

- At first, try taking a bath or shower together and examine each other's genitals. Make sure your partner's genitals are free of bumps, raw redness, or sores. Many STDs can not be seen upon examination, but some, such as genital warts or some herpes sores, can be seen.
- Wear condoms whenever you have penis-vagina, penis-anus, penis-mouth, or vagina-vagina sex.
- Anal sex is more risky.
- After sex, urinate and wash your genitals with warm soapy water to wash out bacterial organisms.
- Don't use IV (intravenous or "shooting up" with a needle) drugs.
- Don't share needles, whether injecting drugs or piercing your body for a tattoo. Make sure all equipment is cleaned and sterilized before using it.
- Never share enemas, douche bags, toothbrushes, or razors with someone.
- Do not share belongings that can have body fluids on them.
- Avoid sex with people who have STDs, prostitutes or IV drug users.
- Assume your sexual partner has a STD and take the appropriate precautions (use a condom or do not exchange body fluids).

## CONTRACEPTION OR BIRTH CONTROL

Contraception and birth control are the same things. These are different ways of preventing or reducing the risk of pregnancy. This section provides an overview of the different types of birth control, how to get them, and information about how to use them. Birth control is not necessarily the same thing as protecting yourself from sexually transmitted diseases. Safe or safer sex will reduce your chances of getting an STD, and birth control will reduce your chances of becoming pregnant if you decide to become sexually active. Knowing your options to prevent pregnancy is very important in avoiding an unplanned pregnancy, and in having to decide how to deal with that issue if you do get pregnant.

## Cheryl's Story: Lost Innocence

Cheryl wrote this story herself, many years after her experience. It is reprinted with her permission, using her own words and voice to tell her story.

> The sun is still sleeping. Its warm fingers will not grace the sky for several hours. I feel cold, although the summer in Mexico City is at its peak. I shiver not from cold but from fear. A dark car approaches the hotel where I stand. The driver moves to open the passenger door. He is well dressed; a white carnation stands in contrast against his black suit. He is the man who will take me away. He beckons me to the car. My body refuses my command to walk. I turn to face my mother. Her smile reaffirms that she loves me. Her eyes try to hide her apprehension. I must go. In the car, I recognize myself in the terrified face of the young girl sitting next to me. I glance out the window to find my mom and wonder if this is the last time I will see her. No one speaks. The silence, like a tomb, encases us as our driver takes us to an unknown location. We travel into the bowels of the city where street vendors prepare for business. I smell tacos frying as dawn brightens the sky. It is the summer of 1970 in Mexico City. I am fifteen years old and I am pregnant.
>
> School is over for the summer. My plans to visit my grandmother in Kentucky are confirmed. I am excited because this is my first time to

travel by plane. I am also burdened with knowing I am pregnant and I have not told anyone, except my boyfriend. "Would my family love me? Perhaps disown me, if they found out? Maybe this will just go away," I keep saying to myself. I ignore the fact that I am sick before I land, blaming the way I feel on the flight. My grandmother, with her warm smile that makes her eyes twinkle with mischief, greets me with a hug. Three days pass and I feel great. I find peace and comfort being here with her. I watch her hands as she sits in her favorite chair. Her glasses, at the tip of her nose, are ready to fall into the mountain of cloth waiting her attention. She takes tiny pieces of fabric, about an inch square, and makes the most beautiful quilts. Hers are kind, gentle hands. The phone rings. My grandmother answers the phone, and with a puzzled look, hands it to me. My heart starts pounding; with dread, I cradle the phone and say hello.

Without a preamble, I hear my mother ask, "Are you pregnant?"

"Yes," I whisper.

"My God, have you thought about what to do?"

"No," I murmur.

How did she find out? She discovered the doctor's receipt while cleaning my room. I thought I threw it away. Subconsciously, I hoped she would find the receipt and help me.

"Cheryl, if you have this child, your life will be ruined. You cannot finish school or enjoy going to the prom. It's the big things and the little things in your life you will miss. You are only fifteen, Cheryl. What do you want to do?"

I can hear the hurt in her voice. I feel ashamed. I know my dad is there and sense his disappointment. "Do they still love me? Am I worthy of their love?" These questions swirl in my brain unanswered.

Pleading for help, I answer, "I don't know, mom."

"We need to make a decision and quickly." Decisive and with purpose, mom takes control. "You must have an abortion. I will make

STDs, Safer Sex, and Birth Control

some calls and call back."

My world is coming undone. Mom makes sense. I am not ready to have a child, but abortion is not legal [it was 1970, and abortion did not become legal in the US until 1973]. Two states, New York and California, have approved abortion; however, the wait is longer than eight weeks. To abort after sixteen weeks is extremely risky. I am fourteen weeks pregnant. I turn to put down the phone.

My grandmother asks, "Cheryl, is everything OK at home?"

"Yes," I say and start to cry.

"You're pregnant, aren't you?" she asks intuitively.

I can only nod my head. I feel like a failure, a disappointment to those I love and who love me.

"Cheryl, these things happen to good girls from the best of families. You are a good girl. Mistakes happen. What are you going to do?"

I explain the option of abortion and that mom will call back. I surrender in my grandmother's open arms and I cry. She holds me close and I breathe deeply, filling my lungs with her essence. I am safe. I wait for THE CALL, bringing information, which will change my life.

My mother contacts her brother in Atlanta. He is a writer for the Atlanta newspaper and is researching an article on abortion. He has information on a group in Mexico City who performs abortions. He arranges for my mother and me to meet in Atlanta. Everything is happening so fast. My uncle contacts someone in Mexico City. According to their instructions, I am to take one only one bag and must travel alone. I will be there in less than twenty-four hours. My mother insists that she travel with me and we book our flight. Arriving in Mexico City, we hail a cab and give the driver the name of the first hotel. There is a list of hotels for us to check. If the first hotel is full, we are to go on to the next one on the list. After checking in, I have a number to call. Following their strict rules, I use an outside pay phone to receive further instructions. First, they tell me no food or water after midnight. The next set of instructions is the most frightening. At 5:00 a.m., a black sedan will pull up in front of the hotel. The driver will wear a carnation in his lapel and take me to an unknown location. I am to be outside waiting. I am not to carry anything with me. I will return that evening in time to catch the flight home. Mystery and foreboding hang heavy in the air. Mom, always the practical one, suggests we eat. As we walk to a nearby restaurant, the smell of taco grease permeates our surroundings. We return to the hotel in silence. I contemplate the illegal abortion. The lights blink outside the room's window. My eyes stare as the colors change the room from gold to red. Sleep eludes my body. I lay in bed anticipating tomorrow.

Although twenty-seven years have passed, the smell of taco grease continues to remind me of my lost innocence. I grew up that summer. I realized the importance of my family. The decision to abort was not easy. Abortion is a personal decision and a personal choice. Nevertheless, the emotional burden on my family and myself brought us closer together. I struggled with my choice for some time. However, I made the right decision. My family supported me and I was fortunate. Many girls faced with this situation have no one to turn to. My experience of having an illegal abortion was successful. Others were not so lucky. Back alley abortions were unsanitary and extremely risky. Thankfully, women no longer have to go underground for an illegal abortion. Today, several help groups provide counseling, education, and birth control to young girls. Through these programs, women do not have to feel alone or unloved. My fear was that my family would disown me. That fear came from the insecurity of a young girl. A young girl who thought she was an adult but was only a child.

189

Cheryl was very fortunate to have a loving, supportive family to help her deal with a very difficult situation. To me, one of the most touching parts of her story is her grandmother telling her that, "These things happen to good girls from the best of families. You are

STDs, Safer Sex, and Birth Control

a good girl." What happened to Cheryl was a mistake. Good people make mistakes, too.

Cheryl was also fortunate to have a caring boyfriend, who she did not mention, but he was supportive. He was her boyfriend for several years through high school. Unfortunately, he really didn't know what to do to help her, and they both buried their heads in the sand about the pregnancy at first. Cheryl was lucky to have parents and a boyfriend who ultimately helped her. Her boyfriend's parents even paid half of the expenses of her travel and abortion.

Cheryl never did not have any other pregnancies. In her twenties, she had health problems unrelated to the abortion and had to have a complete hysterectomy, which is a medical procedure to remove a woman's reproductive organs. While she does believe she made the right decision at the time, she suffered sadness and felt a loss at not experiencing parenthood. Most women think they will have many opportunities for pregnancy and parenthood, but some do not.

Even though abortions are legal today in the United States, an unplanned pregnancy for a teenager still holds many of the same dilemmas that Cheryl faced. The biggest one is: "Will my family still love me? Will they reject me or be supportive? How will I deal with their disappointment?" When Cheryl returned from Mexico, her father had made a banner that he placed across the front door, stating, "Welcome Home, Cheryl." When she saw it, she knew it was going to be OK, even with her father. Yet, for many young women, the fear of facing their parents, family or friends is frightening. Every month, the newspapers report on a young infant that is abandoned and dies in America. Not long ago, a young woman gave birth to a baby in a high school bathroom at her high school prom. She was too afraid to tell her family, and the baby died.

Many times, young women underestimate the ability of parents to set aside their typical conflicts with their children, as well as their personal values, and support their teenagers when an unplanned pregnancy happens. Over and over again, I have witnessed parents who had experienced extensive conflicts with their teenagers rally to support them. One exceptional case was a minister who was the father of a 14 year-old girl. The father was a "pro-lifer" and had participated in demonstrations against abortions. However, when his own young daughter was pregnant, he supported her and her wishes to have an abortion, given the circumstances of her pregnancy. If possible, consider giving your parents a chance to be there for you, even if you are very scared.

Of course, abortion is not the ONLY option to an unplanned pregnancy. In many cases, it is never an option, for whatever individual personal or spiritual reasons. Review Chapter 4, question 7, and consider at length the four options of dealing with pregnancy.

## Four Options for Dealing with an Unexpected Pregnancy

1. Have the baby and keep it to raise yourself.

2. Have the baby and make a plan for adoption.

3. Have the baby and get married or live with the father.

4. Have an abortion.

## GUYS, BIRTH CONTROL, STDS, AND PREGNANCY

Both girls and guys are responsible for planning for birth control and preventing STDs and pregnancy. Unfortunately, as was discussed in Chapter 2, no matter how educated and liberated guys are, many of them are very interested in having sexual relations with girls, but they leave the birth control and STD prevention up to the girl. In fact, some guys take pride in saying, "I will never wear a condom."

Let's face it: pregnancy happens to girls. A pregnancy will not change a guy's life in the same way as it will change *your* life, sometimes forever. Perhaps that's why guys often do not take birth control as seriously as you need to. Men are responsible for paying for child support until a child is 18, out of college, or for a longer period of time if the child is disabled, and support enforcement is getting better, not allowing men to get away with not paying. However, some teenage girls don't want to go for child support, because they are afraid it will make their boyfriend get mad or break up with them. The bottom line is that, if you get pregnant, you will be responsible for caring for the child 24 hours a day, seven days a week, even if you live with your parents. Teenage pregnancy is a difficult situation to handle, even when you have a supportive family or friends.

Prior to 1973, when abortion was legalized, many girls like Cheryl had illegal abortions. Illegal abortions were frightening, life threatening, and expensive for women. Before abortion was legalized, a man who made a woman pregnant was expected to care for her, the baby, and usually marry the woman. In some cases, because of the embarrassment the family felt over a pregnancy outside of marriage, a girl went away to a relative's home in a far away state and gave the baby up for adoption. Often girls who give up their children for adoption live every day wondering if they made the right choice or what happened to their child, or sometimes they feel a sense of loss, even if they knew they made the right decision.

My opinion is that the legalization of abortion gave men an out regarding their responsibility for sex and pregnancy. "Shotgun weddings," where a pregnant girl's father, brother, or uncle threatened a guy with a bodily harm or death, forcing the man to marry her and "do right," defended a woman's honor and made a man responsible for his child. Who knows how good many of those marriages were or if they lasted. Yet, nowadays, many young men feel very little obligation to participate in fatherhood, unless they are legally forced to by a court action. Many young men feel a woman could or should have an abortion or that she should give the baby up for adoption; if she doesn't, he gets mad and often ends the relationship, wanting little to do with a pregnant girlfriend or a child.

VIRGIN SEX *for Girls*

Many guys expect girls to take care of the birth control, then "take care of it" if they are pregnant. Guys haven't changed much: often, they still do not want the responsibility of the potential consequences of sex, which includes the risk of pregnancy. They may not even be involved in the child's life, or they may be involved on a limited basis and with resentment. Sometimes young men are delighted at such a pregnancy and take pride in their manhood, bragging that they are fathers, but most still don't help out or take real responsibility for their children on a daily basis. Often, this causes years of problems for the mother and the child. Granted, many young men take responsibility for their children, and do so lovingly and joyfully with their girlfriends, but that option is the exception.

One of the most difficult things for a girl who has an unplanned pregnancy is telling her boyfriend and awaiting his response. A guy's reaction to an unplanned pregnancy can range from him being supportive, to the absurd, or to the cruel.

## GUYS REACTIONS TO UNPLANNED PREGNANCY

*Supportive*

**"What would YOU like to do?"**
**"How do you FEEL?"**
**"Let's talk to our parents together."**

Some guys, although they are the minority, are supportive, loving, and accept their responsibility in pregnancy. Some guys will really talk to you about how to make a decision to deal with an unplanned pregnancy. Some guys will want you to have the baby, though, when you don't want to: sometimes it is because his parents want you to have the baby because they want custody of the child. With few exceptions, it is the woman's right to decide whether or not to have an abortion, regardless of the father's wishes.

STDs, Safer Sex, and Birth Control

## Denial

"How do I know it's mine?"

"It couldn't be my baby!"

"Are you sure I'm the father? Who have you been messing with?"

Usually a guy's friends and family members tend to support this type of reaction, because of their own denial. Denial, when you KNOW it's his baby, can feel cruel and like rejection. However, it is important to make sure you are confronting the right boy or man as well. Blood tests and DNA testing, in cases of uncertain paternity, can determine who is the father, both before and after a baby is born.

## Abandonment

"If you have the baby, I won't have anything to do with you."

"Well, you're on your own."

"I don't think I want to see you anymore." (Or they just stop calling and coming around.)

"I'm not paying for this baby."

Sometimes, abandonment is just a guy being scared or making threats to you because he wants you to have an abortion. Some guys change their minds after they've gotten over the initial shock. Sometimes a guy means it. It doesn't matter whether this is merely a result of the initial shock or something worse, however, this type of response to your positive pregnancy test can make you feel very alone and scared about handling a pregnancy by yourself.

## Refusal to support you

"I'm never going to pay for that baby."

"You're the one who wanted it. YOU pay for the diapers, clothes, formula, etc . . . ”

**"I'm not paying for an abortion, when I don't really even know if it's mine."**

Very often guys and young men will just assume that if you get pregnant you'll get an abortion, because they don't want the responsibility of having a child. If they want you to have an abortion and you don't, they probably won't stand by you and you'll get emotionally rejected. Do seek support from your family, friends, church or community organizations that help unwed or single mothers.

## Methods of Birth Control

There are a lot of different types of birth control available to women to prevent pregnancy. This section describes different types of birth control, and also tells approximately how effective each type is when used. Effectiveness is how well birth control will protect you against pregnancy. The effectiveness of a birth control method is an approximation, or an estimate, based on how well it works for many women, depending on how well the birth control method is actually used. There are two different rates of effectiveness for birth control: "typical use" and "perfect use." Typical use means how the birth control method is usually used by real people in real situations. Perfect use is the effectiveness of a birth control method when it is used EACH AND EVERY TIME IN THE CORRECT WAY, exactly how it is supposed to be used. For each birth control method, a statistic will be given for how many women get pregnant each year for every 100 women using that method of birth control (Planned Parenthood, 1999). For example, with male condoms, when they are used "perfectly," they are 97% effective. This means that in one year, 3% or 3 women in 100 will become pregnant each year. However, with "typical use" condoms are 86% effective, meaning 14 out of 100 women will get pregnant each year, using this birth control method.

Some types of birth control are available at any local drugstore or the local health department. Some types of birth control require a doctor's prescription. To get a doctor's prescription, you will need to have a "gynecological exam," which is a special type of medical examination from a doctor. When you become sexually active, it is often a good idea to have your first gynecological exam. If you are not sexually active, it is recommended that women have their first gynecological exam when they are 18 years old. A "gynecologist" is a medical doctor who specializes in the treatment of a woman's reproductive system. You don't necessarily have to see a specialist, such as a gynecologist. You can go to a general doctor, visit a women's or teen's health clinic, such as Planned Parenthood, or go the health clinic at college. You may be able to see your pediatrician, if you are under 19. You can also go to your local county health department in some states for a free examination and birth control, from a nurse or doctor.

## The Gynecological Exam

In a gynecological exam, also called a "pelvic exam," a doctor or nurse will examine your genitals, the inside of your vagina, your abdominal region, your rectum and your breasts. A nurse or attendant will always be present while a doctor is doing an exam: it is the law in most states. In order to be examined, you will need to undress, wearing only a doctor's office-provided "gown" to cover mostly the front of you until you are examined. Before the exam, the nurse or doctor will ask you some general health questions, like if you take medication or have any chronic illnesses. During the exam, you will lie down on your back on the doctor's examination table, move your rear end to the very end of the table, and place your feet in "stirrups." Stirrups are metal footholds, which are placed about 2 feet apart in order to place your legs apart to allow the doctor to examine your pelvic area up close. The doctor will lift the bottom of your gown to view your genitals.

Next, the doctor will use a small tool called a "speculum," which is made out of steel and nicknamed "the duck bill." The speculum looks like a small duck bill with a handle, and it opens like a duck's bill to allow the doctor to look inside of your vagina. The speculum is put inside your vagina, with the inserted part being about 5 inches long, so that the inside of your vagina can be clearly seen. First the doctor or the nurse will visually inspect the skin inside of your vagina to make sure it looks the right color and is free of any bumps or sores. The doctor will then take a long "Q-tip" and gently rub it against your cervix, a part of you at the end of your vagina, to get a "swab" of skin cells for microscopic inspection. This skin sample is to test for any problems with the cells inside your vagina, like sexually transmitted diseases or cancer. Next, the doctor will put his finger inside of your vagina to feel your ovaries and make sure they are normal and the right size. The doctor will also feel your abdomen to examine your ovaries and uterus from the outside, to check for normal size and make sure there is no abnormal tenderness.

During a complete gynecological exam, a doctor or a nurse might also do a rectal exam, putting a finger inside your rectum or anus to make sure everything is normal and often feeling your internal organs through your rectum. In addition, after the pelvic examination, a doctor or a nurse will do a breast exam, checking your breasts for any lumps or abnormalities. This means a doctor will feel your breasts, using his or her hands, usually rotating his or her fingers against your chest, feeling for any lumps that could be dangerous to your health.

What is your reaction to reading about a gynecological exam? Even though all women will eventually need to have a gynecological exam, most girls feel afraid or embarrassed by their first gynecological exam. You should always tell a doctor if you feel this way when it is time for your first gynecological exam so that he or she can help prepare you for the new procedure. Remember, however, even if a doctor is absolutely wonderful with you, most women feel somewhat awkward during this procedure. Some women get used to it, others never do; but it is a must for women to have an exam once a year.

> You need to think about whether or not you are prepared to have a gynecological exam, as a part of your decision to be sexually active.

### No Method of Birth Control

When no method of birth control is used, 85–90% of sexually active girls will become pregnant in one year. This means that in any given year, up to 90 girls out of 100 girls who do not use any type of birth control will become pregnant.

### Abstinence

Abstinence is simply not having sexual intercourse, ever and under any circumstances. Pregnancy can't happen if sperm is kept out of your vagina. My dad's entire sex talk was, "Abstinence is the only 100% sure way to prevent pregnancy." He was right. Perfect use of abstinence for birth control has a 0% pregnancy rate, but abstinence must be used each and every time to be effective. "Periodic abstinence" is more commonly or typically used for birth control. Periodic abstinence means that even though people vow that they will not have sex, the vow of abstinence, such as the vow of abstinence from smoking or drinking or speeding, is typically broken with alarming frequency. When one doesn't expect to have sex and uses this as their only birth control method, with no back up method, the failure rate for this method is 20%. Periodic abstinence means that 20 percent of girls who use this as their only means of birth control will become pregnant in one year.

## Outercourse

"Outercourse" is sexual play that does not involve penis-vagina or anal intercourse. Sex play may include vaginal, oral or anal sexual stimulation. Outercourse is nearly 100% effective in preventing pregnancy. Pregnancy is still possible if semen or "pre-ejaculate" contacts the vulva (this could happen even in anal intercourse), however, and the sperm can swim inside the vagina. Pre-ejaculate is a small amount of semen that is discharged from the penis when a guy gets excited but hasn't yet ejaculated or come, so merely stopping before he ejaculates is not necessarily an effective method of avoiding pregnancy. Outercourse is effective against HIV and STDs as well unless bodily fluids are exchanged through oral or anal sex or by skin-to-skin contact through small, even microscopic, cuts or openings of the skins, such as blisters or sores.

## The Pill

The birth control pill is the most popular method of birth control for teenagers. A gynecological exam is necessary and a prescription for pills is required. Some health insurance plans pay for birth control pills, and many women's clinics give them away for free. The pill is a hormone used to prevent ovulation, so that pregnancy is not possible. It is a highly effective method of birth control, when used consistently and correctly. Some women have side effects from hormones and can't take the pill, so they need to talk to their health care professional about this. The birth control patch and ring work in similar hormonal ways as the pill, although they put the hormones in your body differently. Talk to your health care professional to see if these options are right for you. With perfect use, the pill is 99.5% effective. Typical use has 95% effectiveness.

### Condoms

Condoms are available over the counter at drug stores, some super-markets, women's clinics, the local health clinic and even Wal-Mart. The condom is called a "barrier" method of birth control, mean-ing there is a barrier preventing sperm from fertilizing the egg and causing pregnancy. A condom is a sheath, like a fitted balloon that covers the penis, made of latex, plastic, or animal tissue. Condoms, when used consistently, can be highly effective in preventing preg-nancy and protect against STDs. Female condoms are shaped to fit inside a woman's vagina and protect against pregnancy and STDs in the same manner, by providing a barrier to keep sperm from fer-tilizing the egg. Female condoms can be used for heterosexual or homosexual sexual activities. Male condoms with perfect use have 97% effectiveness: however, typical use effectiveness is 86%.

200

### Diaphragm and Cervical Cap

These two birth control devices are obtained by prescription, from a doctor or nurse practitioner, following a gynecological exam. You only have to go to a clinic or doctor's office once to get one. It is a "barrier" method made of latex, and it is specifically fitted to your size. These devices are inserted into your vagina and fit over your cervix. They block semen from entering your uterus, with the help of spermicidal jelly. A diaphragm or cervical cap can be used over and over again. These devices are fitted for a woman by a doctor so that they will fit the woman's individual cervix size (and there are many different sizes). These devices are used with a spermicidal jelly, which kills sperm. Most pregnancies occur with these devices because a woman doesn't know a spermicidal jelly has to be used with it every time. Most commonly, in the passion of the sexual moment, one of these devices is simply not used. A diaphragm and cervical cap must be used each and every time sexual intercourse occurs to be effective. Perfect use is 96% effective for a diaphragm, and 94% effective for a cervical cap. Typical use is 81% effective for a diaphragm and 80% effective for a cervical cap. As you can see, these methods can be highly effective when used all the time and correctly, but have a failure rate, or pregnancy rate when they are not used all the time.

### Intrauterine Device or IUD

An IUD, or intrauterine device, must be obtained by prescription from doctor or nurse practitioner, and the prescription is followed by gynecological exam. An IUD is a small plastic device fitted and placed inside a woman's uterus. It can be left in place 5–10 years, but it needs to be checked at least every two years. An IUD is the world's most frequently used reversible method of birth control. It works by not allowing the egg to implant on the uterine wall. It is not intended for teenagers to use—it is generally recommended for women in monogamous relationships who already have children, as some women can in rare situations develop infections and sterility. Perfect and typical uses of an IUD device are both close to 99% effectiveness.

### Contraceptive foams, gels, and suppositories

All of these methods are available without a doctor or nurse's prescription from a drug store or grocery store. All of these methods work as spermicides, which means they kill sperm. When used alone, these methods are about as effective as condoms. Used with condoms, they are 99% effective and nearly as effective as the pill! The use of condoms and spermicides, when used together and used each and every time, are highly effective in preventing pregnancy, and you can easily get these at your local grocery or drug store, without having to go to a doctor or get a prescription, making this method of birth control easily accessible for young women.

Some women may have an allergic reaction or irritation from latex or certain types of spermicides. Changing your brand may solve the problem. On the lighter side, one girl shared a funny story about contraceptive foam, saying it worked fine, but it made noises during sex because of the "foaminess" with the vaginal lubrication, making sounds during intercourse like a churning washing machine.

### Norplant

Norplant used to be obtained from a doctor or nurse following a gynecological exam. A six-capsule hormonal implant was inserted under the skin of the upper arm. Like the pill, this method of birth control was reversible, but it had to be removed from under your skin. It was removed from the U.S. market in 2002. However, as its effects last for five years, some implants may be in circulation still.

### Depo-Provera

Depo-Provera is an injectable hormone that lasts 12 weeks. You have to get an exam and see a doctor or nurse, who will give you a shot in your arm. This method is a very effective and convenient method of birth control. It affects your body like the pill, preventing you from ovulating, so you can't get pregnant. The advantage to Depo-Provera shots is that you don't have to remember to take a pill every day, and you just have to go to the doctor or clinic once every 3 months. There may be side effects, however, as with all birth control pills, and a negative aspect is that there is no way to stop the possible side effects until the shot wears off in 12–14 weeks. For some girls, it is a good idea to try birth control pills first to see if you have any negative side effects before going on Depo shots.

## Withdrawal

Withdrawal is also known as "pulling out." Pulling out or withdrawing means a guy removes his penis from your vagina just prior to ejaculating his semen when he has an orgasm. Used perfectly, withdrawal has an effectiveness rate of 96%. Typical use of withdrawal has an 81% effectiveness rate. That means that in one year, using withdrawal, 19 girls out of 100 will get pregnant every year. Withdrawal is a very risky method of birth control for young people. Mostly, this is due to young men often having poor control over their ability to control their ejaculation. Basically, many young men do not know exactly when they are going to come or how fast they will come and predicting the moment to pull out can be very tricky and unreliable. The withdrawal method is better than using no method of birth control at all, but it is a very risky method of birth control for preventing pregnancy for young women.

203

## Emergency Contraception

This is commonly called "the morning after pill." This is an available method for women if contraception fails, like if a condom breaks, if you are raped, or if any type of unexpected unprotected sex takes place. It is very effective if taken within 72 hours of unprotected sex. Sometimes, a woman has to go to a health clinic or doctor's office to receive this treatment. In some states, it is available directly from a pharmacy, just by asking the pharmacist for the medication. Although in some states where it is legal to obtain emergency contraception from a pharmacy, some pharmacies, due to their ethical beliefs, that using it is similar to having a very early abortion, will not carry it. If one doesn't have it, try another pharmacy, or call around to find a pharmacy which does keep this pill in stock. This method does not protect a girl from STDs, but it does prevent pregnancy.

## Sterilization

Sterilization is the most widely used form of birth control, but it is almost always reserved for men and women who are much older, and it is almost always inappropriate for teenagers. Sterilization is a permanent surgical procedure to prevent pregnancy, and it is frequently irreversible. You shouldn't even think about getting sterilized or agree that your partner undergo sterilization until you are absolutely certain that you do not want any more children; most doctors will not perform this surgery until you have had children and/or you are well over 30 years old. Sterilization may be possible to reverse in some cases, but the procedure is very expensive and reversals only work 25% of the time. "Vasectomy" is the terms for a man's sterilization procedure. This is where the tubes that carry sperm for ejaculation are permanently cut and blocked. "Tubal ligation" is the terms for women's sterilization. This is where the tubes that carry eggs, the fallopian tubes, are cut and blocked.

## Natural Family Planning

Also called fertility awareness methods, these methods do not involve pills or devices. Natural family planning includes several different methods, which are most effective when used together. These methods are called: post ovulation, cervical mucous or ovulation, calendar or rhythm, and thermal or basal body temperature. A fertile woman's body gives off subtle signs of fertility during the menstrual cycle which can be tracked to determine when a woman will get pregnant. These methods have a relatively high failure rate, and require a great deal of responsibility to be used correctly. It is highly recommended that if you choose these methods, you obtain detailed instruction and information from a health care educator concerning proper use. Since teenagers often have irregular periods, it is recommended that you consider other methods of birth control. Typical use of natural family planning methods have 90–99% effectiveness rates.

# *nine*

# PURE VIRGIN SEX

206

Virgin sex should be pure and not dirty or bad or painful. Sex for the first time can be a positive, joyful experience, rather than tainted with pain that sometimes lasts many years. Emotionally and physically, sex can be either painful or joyful, depending on whether or not you are ready for the experience.

Some parents want you to experience sexual relationships only when you are married, so it will be special, sharing sex with only one person in your life. Most parents want you to delay sex until you are "older," so that you can fully understand the responsibilities of sexual relationships. In reality, a minority of people today are virgins when they get married. In fact, the majority of teenagers have their first sexual experiences, including sexual intercourse, before they finish high school. Unfortunately, because many parents and adults want to encourage sexual abstinence, they may not talk to you specifically about sexual relationships at a time when you need the information the most: when you are a virgin and beginning to have your first sexual experiences, especially if these things occur when you are still a teenager and particularly vulnerable to misinformation and when you are faced with more difficult choices than you ever have been before. As a result, most teenagers have no sexual education that specifically addresses both the emotional and physical parts of sexual relationships, especially virgin sex. Perhaps this is why your parents may have helped you lay your hands on this book: to help you make the best decision for yourself sexually and to help you avoid getting hurt from sex.

Virgin Sex does not encourage or promote sexual relationships outside marriage or when you are a teenager. It does provide information for teens and young adults who choose to have sexual experiences with knowledge that may be difficult or impossible to receive at home or at school. Simply put, this information is important if you are to have initial sexual experiences that do not hurt you, emotionally or physically. You may want to share this chapter with your boyfriend, so you can talk about your thoughts and feelings together, as well as your values and desires when it comes to sexual feelings and experiences. The overall goal is to help you make the best decisions about sex for yourself and for each other.

207

## PART I: THE EMOTIONAL SIDE OF SEX

Your emotions are your feelings. Sex can make you feel good, but it can also make you feel very bad. Sex can be one of the greatest joys on earth, but it can make you feel deeply regretful and depressed, too. When people get hurt from sex, aside from getting STDs or an unwanted pregnancy, it is usually because their feelings get hurt. Sex can make you feel all mixed up about people, relationships, and life. It is very important to pay attention to the emotional side of sex. The most important thing to remember about avoiding emotional pain is: Only have sex when you are ready in every way.

### Don't just let sex "happen": Be ready for sex

Ask yourself if you are really ready for sex before sex happens. Take the Dr. Darcy's "Am I Ready for Sex?" Quiz (in Chapter 4), whether you are a virgin or if you've already had sexual experiences. Don't just let sex happen and then regret it later. Do your best to make the best decision before you have sex. If you've already had sex for the first time, it's important that you are ready for any new sexual experience, whether you are 12 years old or 70 years old! Every sexual experience is important! Even if you're not a virgin, and regardless of the quality of your previous experiences, deciding who you are today sexually is important for who you will be tomorrow. It is never too late to make a decision about who you are and what you want in any new sexual situation.

~~~~~~~

> It is not important who you were yesterday or last year: The day you start making a decision about what is important for you sexually is the day you become your own sexual person.

~~~~~~~

When you become your own sexual person, you will become more grown up and be more emotionally healthy when it comes to sex. You are the only one who can make this decision: not any guy, not any parent, only you. When you think about and respond emotionally to what you want to do with this special part of your being, at the very least you are being true to yourself. Even if you make a mistake, and everyone has made some mistakes about sex, at least you can rest assured that you have always tried your utmost to be true to yourself. If you suddenly find yourself in a sexual situation and don't have the time to think ahead about sex (or better yet to go back to Chapter 4 and review), take the time to do the following:

## Quick Hits: Two Last Minute Sex Questions

- HOW WILL I FEEL AFTER SEX WITH THIS PERSON?
- HOW WILL I THINK ABOUT MYSELF AFTER SEX?

Really listen to your heart and mind, and pay attention to the answers. One of the biggest emotional mistakes people make when it comes to sex is simply not making that big a deal of it and not thinking ahead about the emotional, physical, and spiritual consequences that accompany sex. Some people fool themselves into believing that "sex is no big deal." Yet, when they look back, they realize it was, but they didn't expect to feel the way that the experience made them feel.

If you are in the middle of a date or in some other sudden sexual situation, try to answer these two last minute questions when you are alone. Get away from your partner for just a few minutes. Find a quiet place to consider your options for a moment. Even if it is a quick escape to the bathroom in the middle of a loud party, give yourself a couple of minutes to think. Close your eyes and be still. Listen to your heart, listen to your mind, listen to your gut, and listen to your body . . . then wait a few seconds for an answer. Do what is right for you, always.

## What Teens Think About Before Sex

Girls and guys both have insecurities about sex, but there are differences in what kind of worries they have before sex. The important thing to remember is to be caring, reassuring, and always keep the lines of sexual communication open before, during and after sex.

## Some Things Guys Think About Before Sex:

- When guys have sex for the first time, they often think, "I feel a special connection and hope she feels a special connection, too!"
- "I'm afraid she might get pregnant!"

- They may think that they just want to lose their virginity, and nothing else matters but feeling the physical experience they have looked forward to for a long time.

- If they have had sex before, with someone else, they may feel some of the same feelings as when they lost their virginity, but there tends to be less searching for the emotional connection with their girlfriend and more interest in the physical pleasures of sex.

- They may ask themselves if they are physically attractive to their girlfriend; however, they are not as worried about physical appearance as girls are. For boys this thought is more like, "Does she think I'm hot?"

- "What does she look like naked?" Most guys are not nearly as concerned about what your body looks like or seeking perfection as the fact that they get to see you and be with you naked.

- Some guys worry about their "performance," or if they have pleased their girlfriend.

- However, some guys are on the quest for YOUR orgasm only in order to prove they're sexual studs.

- They wonder if their penis is big enough or hard enough.

- Guys worry that they will ejaculate too soon.

- Some guys want to make sex last too long, thinking it proves they're sexual studmuffins, without realizing it might not be what you want.

- Some guys may want to prove to themselves that they are not gay.

- Some guys just want to experience sexual control over another person.

# Some Things Girls Think About Before Sex

- Girls worry that sex for the first time will be physically painful.

- Girls worry about pregnancy and STDs and they want protection. A lot of times, they are too afraid to talk about protection, and they want the guy to bring it up.

- Girls tend to need a lot of reassurance from a guy that they are loved and respected. It is important for a girl to feel like she did the right thing. She will know this by how a guy acts not only before sex but also after sex.

- Girls worry about their bodies and if they look good naked. They are worried about being too fat: if their breasts are attractive or too big or too small, if their stomach is flat, or if their butt is OK.

211

- Girls are afraid that they'll get pressured into sex and go farther than they want to go with sexual exploration.

- If sex "just happens" and they didn't talk to the guy about it ahead of time, they tend to have feelings of remorse, sadness, and guilt.

- It is always best for virgin sex to be planned. Girls need to talk about sex and be prepared, emotionally and physically, to share their virginity.

- Girls think about orgasms, although not so much the first time. They wonder if they will have one, how to have one, and what it is like.

- Girls think about the guy's orgasm. They wonder: When will he come and what will it be like?

- On giving oral sex, girls wonder what they're supposed to do when the guy comes: pull off, spit, or swallow?

- On getting oral sex, girls worry if they smell OK (because of all the tasteless jokes and advertisements for feminine hygiene products) and if their partner really wants to do it.

- Girls are not worried about the size of a man's penis, unless it is really too big.

- Some girls get scared when they see an erect penis for the first time and wonder, "How is that big thing going to fit inside of me?"

- Girls want to make sure they are the "only one" and a guy is not just "playin' her" and using her for just sex.

- If a girl is having casual sex, she still wants to feel respected by the guy and know the guy will treat her like a friend afterwards.

## PART II: THE PHYSICAL SIDE OF SEX

### Lisa's Story

Lisa was almost 15 when she had her first sexual experience with a guy. Lisa had been going out with her boyfriend for several months prior to their serious discussion about making love together. "Will" had previously had a sexual relationship with a girl who was a virgin, and he reassured Lisa that they would take it slow so that she wouldn't get hurt.

The two of them had spent a lot of time together, talking about their feelings of love and caring for each other, making out, and discussing the possibility of having a sexual relationship together. Lisa felt ready to make love to Will, but she was afraid of sex hurting because her girlfriends talked about how awful sex was and how much it hurt. After planning out how to proceed, Will got some condoms and told Lisa that they would take it slowly.

Losing her virginity took place over three days. Each time they spent together started out the same way. They talked, hugged each other, kissed and touched, then they proceeded to have sexual contact. The first day, Will just put the head of his penis into Lisa's vagina. He didn't thrust his penis hard into her: he just gently put the tip of his penis inside the lips of her labia and entered her vagina. Lisa felt very good about this intimate contact and actually wanted to go further, but Will told her they would take it slowly. The next time, Will entered her vagina about 2 inches. He did move back and forth, in and out of her vagina slowly, but he only entered her vagina at the most 2 inches at a time. Lisa did not feel any pain, nor did she experience bleeding. In fact, she felt very comfortable and had a desire to go further, but Will urged her to wait, allowing her vagina to get stretched out and used to penetration. He suggested that they wait until the next time they were together. After this initial sexual experimentation, Lisa did not feel physically uncomfortable at all. She felt ready to proceed and to lose her virginity. In reality, she was looking forward to going further and having full intercourse, instead of being afraid.

After a few days, they got together again, made out for a while, then proceeded to "try" to have sex again. This time, Will entered her vagina slowly with his penis and was able to fully place his penis in her vagina. He did not shove it in or thrust back and forth at first; he just went slowly. Lisa did not feel pain, and surprisingly, she does not remember bleeding at all. After this, Will began to move slowly in and out of her in order to have sexual arousal for both of them. According to Lisa, they did not really start having full deep penetration and thrusting for about 2 months. After 2 months, Lisa felt very comfortable with vigorous sexual intercourse.

This story surprised me, as I had never heard of a girl losing her virginity over a period of a week or with three sexual encounters. I was totally surprised that she had a boyfriend who was this patient and smart enough to work with her in losing her virginity in a way that

213

was loving, safe, and pain-free. Lisa dated Will for several months, and their break up, while sad, was on pretty good terms. Lisa says she will always be grateful for Will being such a great guy and will never forget the positive experience of losing her virginity with him.

Interestingly, Lisa is now in a lesbian relationship. She didn't realize until later in her adolescence that she was far more attracted to woman, physically and sexually, than to guys. As she puts it, "It goes to show that not all lesbians are with women because of bad experiences with men." Lisa simply realized she loved women, not that she didn't like men.

## Virgin Sex without Physical Pain

Girls need to be in control of their sexuality to experience virgin sex without getting hurt physically, or at least in order to feel only a degree of physical sexual discomfort. Remember: you are responsible for your own sexuality and young men need to be completely directed by girls, even if they are experienced, for girls to avoid physical pain with sex. The expectation in our culture is that virgin sex will hurt. The urban sexual myth is that guys will be the sexual aggressor, the "experienced" ones, who will know what to do and have control over sex. This is the main reason why virgin sex hurts and it is a bad situation that needs to change.

Guys feel as though they should know exactly what to do in sex, but in reality, they usually don't. In Lisa's story above, her boyfriend, Will, was the exception and a role model for guys who are with virgins or sexually inexperienced girls. Yet, even if a guy knows about how girls "work," exactly what works for any girl on any given day is a mystery and only YOU know the answer to that question. No guy in the world can read a girl's mind (or body) and know everything she wants or likes on any given day. Allowing a guy to decide for you what happens sexually is almost always a mistake that can hurt you. A guy can only know what to do if YOU talk to him. Sexual sharing can only be wonderful if you are willing to share who you are and what you want, what you like and dislike.

# The Three Steps of Virgin Sex

1. Talking and listening
2. Touching and feeling
3. Sexual Touch and Sexual Intercourse

## Talking and Listening

Nowadays, giving a guy oral sex, then the guy trying to "pop your cherry" are often the first two steps of virgin sex. The truth is that the relationship between the couple is the most important first connection for a sexual relationship. Remember, how you feel emotionally toward each other will affect any physical connection. Girls and guys need to evaluate an emotional connection in order to really know if this is the right person, time and place for sex before sharing themselves sexually with someone. The way to tell if you are ready for the first step of virgin sex is if the two of you can talk and listen to each other.

One of the steps you might want to take together as a couple in talking and listening is considering the Dr. Darcy's "Am I Ready for Sex?" Quiz together. You can use this guide to talk about your conditions for sex, to know if you are prepared for some of the physical and emotional consequences of sex, as well as to evaluate other considerations that may be important or personal to you. Become comfortable with sexual communication, using the guide in Chapter 6, to share your sexual thoughts, ideas, needs and feelings.

After talking and listening, ask yourself: **Can I really trust this person?** Review Chapter 5 and think about your relationship with your boyfriend. You have to decide if your boyfriend really likes and respects you, if he will be there for you, if he is telling the truth, and if he can talk to you about how you feel. Guys are different from girls in their emotional needs as related to sex, but that does not mean that they can not be there for you and give you the type of support and concern that you deserve and require as a young woman. If he can't talk to you and listen, especially without jumping into sex first, then he is too immature to have a sexual relationship with you.

Think about your comfort level: If you aren't comfortable emotionally, chances are that you will not feel comfortable sexually either, especially with virgin sex, no matter how much you think you love him.

## Touching and Feeling

For girls to have sex without pain, first they must have sexual desire and sexual arousal. As discussed in more detail in the last chapter, sexual desire is a feeling of "wanting" another person and/or a feeling of horniness. Sexual arousal means feeling sensations of physical excitement or being "turned on." If there is no arousal from sexual desire and a feeling of being excited, it is not a good idea to continue with a sexual relationship. If you are ready for sex, a physical relationship starts with touch.

Some sex therapists consider the skin the largest sex organ, since it covers your whole body. Touch is very powerful physically and emotionally, but it is largely overlooked as it relates to sexual experience unless there is genital contact. Touch can be very exciting, erotic, and even provide deep sexual sensations, but if it does not include genital contact, most people don't think of it as sexual behavior. For example, kissing can be fun, exciting, passionate, intimate, and sexy, but it's not considered sexual, since no sexual parts are touched. Yet, for a lot of girls, deep French kissing is a big turn on and an essential part of foreplay. Giving each other foot rubs or

216

back rubs generally represents totally non-sexual touching, but these things can be big turn-ons for each other too. The most important part of this stage of physical sharing is for you to experience and feel comfortable with physical touch. First, enjoy being physical with a guy in a safe, non-threatening way (which means he's not going to pressure you) that does not include sexual contact. If you do not feel comfortable with this type of physical sharing and experience then you will not enjoy any further sexual contact, either.

Next, see if you feel sexual desire and arousal without sexual touching. If you feel comfortable with your partner, it is very likely that you will feel turned on with non-sexual touch. At this point, it is also the time to be sure that you trust your partner to listen to you and respect your sexual limits, with how fast to go and how far to go with touching. If he doesn't respect your physical and sexual limits with non-sexual touch, he certainly won't pay attention to you and respect you with sexual contact.

> All sexual touch between people needs to be negotiated and agreed upon. This means that each person talks and communicates both verbally and nonverbally, about what each person wants in each and every sexual situation.

## Sexual Touch

Sexual exploration is the third step of virgin sex. Sexual touch, without sexual intercourse, may take place over a very long period of time, especially for sexually inexperienced young women and men. Exploring how one feels and sharing sexual feelings with sexual, non-intercourse touch may occur in a relationship for weeks or months or forever, without ever having sexual intercourse. Many girls save sexual intercourse for marriage or for someone very special, while sharing sexual touch in one or more relationships before losing their virginity.

Usually sexual touch and sexual sharing, even without sexual intercourse, is enjoyable and physically pleasurable for guys and girls.

As stated before, we are wired for sex before birth. Yet, it is important to explore what feels good to you with sexual touch, long before you will feel comfortable with sexual intercourse. Many girls have already experienced sexual touch from masturbation or self-pleasuring. Girls who are experienced with sexual self touch will have a better idea of what to expect with sexual touching of their genitals than girls who have not sexually explored on their own. Yet, sexual touch with a partner is usually a more intense physical experience, because it is combined with excitement of shared emotions and the element of surprise with a partner's touch.

Both of you will want to explore what feels good to you with sexual touch, in both giving and receiving sexual touch. The most important part of this step is to first have sexual exploration without a guy using his penis to give you sexual pleasure; you do not start with sexual intercourse. A guy may use his hands, mouth, or fingers to allow you to feel sexual pleasure, but NEVER start with his penis. The beginning of sexual touch is your partner touching your breasts, buttocks, and genitals, and you touching his body, buttocks, nipples, and genitals, too. Guys are responsible for asking for permission to touch a girl in a sexual area, be it her breasts, buttocks, or genitals, and you need to ask him what is OK, too.

> If you don't want sexual touch: then say "stop," at any point. A guy is responsible for asking you to have sexual touch and how much. Many guys, when they are making the moves on you and you don't say no, will take that as yes and won't stop until you do say no.

For girls, usually the most sexually exciting part of her body is her clitoris. Most inexperienced guys don't know how to touch your clitoris. A lot of guys don't know where the heck a clitoris is, or even what it is, not to mention how to touch it in a way that is enjoyable to you. Typically, most girls, dressed or naked, will experience sexual pleasure with touch to the clitoris. Clitoral touch can be with a leg, pelvis, hand, vibrator, mouth or tongue. Generally, clitoral stimulation involves rubbing your clitoris in and up and down, back and forth, or with a pressing motion, depending on what you like. You need to guide your partner with directions, and you can start by saying: higher, lower, faster, slower or softer or harder. In some cases, you might put your hand on his and guide him with the motions that are pleasurable and exciting to you.

Next, girls need to know what guys need, too. First, this step involves a guy showing his penis to a girl. When a guy is not sexually excited, his penis is soft or "flaccid" and may be big or small, but the size of a flaccid penis does not always predict its size when the guy is aroused. When a guy is sexually excited, he gets an erection, or a "hard-on," and his penis is hard and bigger than when flaccid. A guy needs to tell a girl how to touch his penis, and if she wants to, to kiss it and suck it (no teeth!). Guys also need to show you how to touch their testicles: with what firmness, how to pull them, squeeze them, rub them, or suck on them. As with girls, sexual touch with a guy may start with a hand. Touching a guy's penis with your hand involves touching or stroking. Vigorous stroking of the penis—using an up and down motion with your hand holding the penis firmly— to the point of orgasm is called a "hand job."

Most guys will try to touch you or try to "get farther" with you by rushing touch with their hands or mouth. Even though they are supposed to ask first, when you're making out, you might just start touching each other without talking about it. However, you need to take direct responsibility for your sexuality by **saying** yes or no, and guiding (OR PUSHING AWAY) a guy as you so desire. Girls need to clearly SAY what they mean, not just motion with their hands or body or looks, to let a guy know how far they can go. You need to tell guys with your voice how far you want them to go **before** you have sexual intercourse. You need to let a guy know if you just want to hug and kiss, touch, or something more.

> A word of caution: If you get into a lot of sexual touch, most guys, and a lot of girls, are going to get excited and want sex immediately.

Remember, a guy's sexual drive is incredibly powerful. A mature guy will have will power and patience with you, putting aside his immediate needs for sexual release and satisfaction, even if you are touching him or visa versa with sexual exploration. If he can't do that, he is not the guy for you. He is not sexually safe and trustworthy, and he needs to work seriously on his self-control skills and spend more time in a cold shower. Yet, it is wise to think responsibly about how you or a guy might be getting excited as you progress with sexual touch. If you are feeling strongly about not having sexual intercourse, you need to tell him up front. As much as you are not responsible for his sexual feelings, if you don't tell him before sexual exploration or big-time making out, he might think you're a "tease," or a "dick-tease." You may want to consider limiting messing around to non-sexual touch like kissing or hugging and not letting things get too hot and heavy, if you discover that you definitely do not want a sexual relationship of any kind.

## ORAL SEX

Oral sex is touching someone's genitals with your mouth, and it is also called "giving head," or on guys, "giving a blow job." Some people like this, while others don't. For guys and girls, please remember that oral sex is a risky sexual behavior, since it involves the transmission of sexual fluids from the genitals to the mouth (see Chapter 8 on STDs). On the other hand, one of the great things about oral sex is that you can share love and intimacy and you will not get pregnant. Currently, oral sex is a very popular type of non-intercourse sex between teenagers, especially with girls giving blowjobs to guys.

A lot of girls and guys don't seem to think that oral sex "counts" as sex, but if you are having sexual touch of any kind, it's sex. If someone comes, it's sex. If sexual fluids are exchanged at all, it's sex. Some girls give guys blowjobs because it takes sexual pressure off of them; they can get a guy off without "having to have sex." Interestingly, recent research on teens and oral sex show that about 50% of teen guys and girls are both giving and receiving oral sex; however, 70% of teen guys report receiving oral sex, while only 50% report giving oral sex (Mosher et al, 2002). With half of teens experiencing oral sex, it is very important to remember that any sexual contact requires the use of safe protection against STDs. Oral sex on a guy can occur with the use of condoms, including flavored condoms, such as fruit or mint flavors, to protect girls from sexually transmitted infections.

## ANAL SEX

Anal sex refers to sexual contact with the anus, which is commonly referred to as your "butthole." Anal sex can involve any stimulation of the anus, including touching, licking, or anal penetration. For some people, the anus is a highly sensitive area, bringing intense sexual pleasure, although many people feel "grossed out" by any anal contact. Touching may include touching with a hand or an object, such as tickling with a feather. Anal touching with a mouth may be as simple as kissing and touching the area around the anus. Actually licking the anus for sexual play is called "rimming." Rimming is unsafe sex, and a latex barrier or part of a condom needs to be used to have safer sex. If you don't want to have anal sex, but your boyfriend insists on it, you might try joking with him, sarcastically saying, "We can have anal sex any time *you* want to: Just bend over."

The opening of the anus has a sphincter, which is less elastic than a vagina. For this reason, sexual penetration needs to begin very slowly, or it may be the first and last experience with anal sex you ever have. You need to learn relaxation, and you need a lot of lubrication. For most people, it takes days, weeks, or months for the anal sphincter to stretch out and be prepared for anal penetration. Anal penetration can begin with a tongue or finger, and may progress to using a small, slender object or anal dildo, or a penis. Some teenagers choose to engage in anal sex for experimentation, to enjoy sexual variation and pleasure, to have sexual intercourse during a woman's period, or to maintain a girl's technical virginity by leaving the vaginal hymen intact; but one of the biggest reasons for teenagers to have anal sex is to avoid the risk of pregnancy that accompanies vaginal intercourse. It is important to know that anal sex still carries the risk of STDs, especially Hepatitis B, and all sexual precautions need to be taken. Some people never learn to enjoy anal sex and/or have no interest in this type of sexual experimentation, however, anal sex, or "buggery" as it used to be called, is also illegal in several states.

With anal sex, it is essential that you trust your partner to be gentle and that you feel very comfortable using your sexual voice to say what you want. You have to listen to your body and be heard when you say stop.

## SEXUAL INTERCOURSE

Prior to sexual intercourse, after "foreplay" or sexual touch, sexual exploration of vaginal penetration with a finger or tongue first is the best way to prepare for pain-free sexual intercourse. A tongue or finger is much smaller, and less scary and intimidating, than a penis for most girls. For one thing, you can't get pregnant with a tongue or finger. For another, the tongue or finger is less wide and long, and it usually won't be uncomfortable if penetration is started slowly. For virgins, the use of a tongue or finger can introduce sexual pleasure along with vaginal penetration.

In my opinion, it is preferable for women to experience orgasm prior to sexual intercourse. An orgasm occurs from intense sexual excitement, meaning a girl is more sexually aroused and more likely to have vaginal lubrication that allows for easier sexual intercourse. When a girl is sexually aroused, her vagina expands and lengthens about 2 inches longer, making sexual penetration possible, less painful, and more naturally easier. If a girl is not physically aroused, and her vagina has not lengthened, she can experience pain from a man's penis hitting the "back of her vagina," or against her cervix. Also, a woman's pain tolerance increases with sexual excitement and arousal, so any concerns of sexual discomfort with intercourse decrease, too, making intercourse, especially for virgin sex, more comfortable, less painful, or even pain-free. Ideally, a young woman can explore her own body with self touch, learn what turns her on, and guide her partner into giving her sexual pleasure. Experiencing sexual excitement and/or orgasm prior to intercourse makes sexual intercourse more physically comfortable and pleasurable, and it is more likely that you will experience an orgasm during intercourse, increasing sexual pleasure. For pain-free, comfortable and enjoyable sex, it is best to delay vaginal penetration until you have had at least several experiences with sexual touch and exploration, preferably learning how to have an orgasm, whether it is clitoral and/or vaginal orgasms. Of course, not all women are able to experience orgasms, but being physically sexually excited, and having vaginal lubrication and wetness is necessary for comfortable and pleasurable sexual intercourse, at all times.

If you have sexual touch and do not respond with sexual excitement, you are not ready for sexual intercourse. A number of factors may cause a lack of sexual excitement, but a lack of arousal usually means that you are not prepared for vaginal penetration, emotionally and physically. Go back to Chapter 4 and see if you are ready for sex. For example, one of your "conditions" for sex might be that you need to be in love, and if you're not, you aren't able to respond with excitement to sexual touch. Turn to Chapter 5 and evaluate whether or not you can trust your partner and/or if you think he likes you. Read the section in Chapter 7 on sexual arousal. Review the section on "Sex for One" in Chapter 7 to learn about your own sexual responses to help you prepare for shared sexual expression.

> If you do not respond to sexual touch with physical excitement and arousal, you are not ready for sexual intercourse, and you can hurt yourself, emotionally and/or physically.

Any person who just wants to "ram it in there" is the wrong person to share sex with, and he is probably a lousy sexual partner, too. You need someone who will start slowly and be patient with YOUR needs, whether you are a virgin or sexually experienced. Movies that show people slamming against a wall, then frantically roving each others' bodies with their hands, quickly progressing to the genital area followed by falling on a bed or couch and instant sexual intercourse, are not demonstrations of how to have pleasurable virgin sex. Hollywood sex may be great for a couple with a trusting, established sexual relationship, but it's a myth that women want or need this type of sexual forcefulness and it can hurt a virgin or young, inexperienced woman.

Vaginal penetration can be pleasurable or invasive. A young woman needs to be in control of what is put inside her vagina: how far, how fast, and how long. You need to make this decision for yourself, with the thoughts in your mind and the feelings from your body as the basis for your decision. A guy just reaching as far as he can into your pants and getting what he can, even by putting only his finger inside you, can feel like a sexual violation. It is a sexual violation if you didn't agree to it. Rushed, or even forced, genital touch, and especially vaginal penetration, makes a girl turned off to sexual intercourse, sometimes with long lasting effects. Besides, if you are not sexually turned on or your vagina is dry, it can be physically painful.

For many young women, sexual playfulness that starts with touch and sexual exploration, followed with vaginal penetration by a tongue or finger, slowly, is usually sexually exciting. Prior to penetration, lubrication of the vagina and penis is essential. Usually, with sexual excitement, a girl's vagina will be wet and moist inside through natural lubrication. If there is no wetness, or if it decreases with sexual activity, an over-the-counter lubricant, such as *Astroglide, K-Y jelly*, or *WET*, will work (don't use regular hand lotion, which will cause dryness or harm the skin over time). Saliva is a great lubricant and is easily available.

At first, just find the vaginal opening and see how it feels to have a finger slowly and simply placed inside of you. Watch out for long or sharp fingernails, which will poke you. Start with exploring how deeply you feel comfortable with penetration, reaching as far inside your vagina toward your cervix, which feels firm and has a semi-circular shape, as you feel comfortable. After you feel comfortable with finger insertion, venture on to moving the finger back and forth and around against the walls of the vagina, then in and out of the vagina, not quite removing the finger fully out of the vagina. It is important with virgin sex, and first sexual experiences, to have the vagina get comfortable with penetration and to gently stretch the vaginal opening in preparation for sexual intercourse.

.Sexual exploration of vaginal penetration with a finger or tongue needs to be a process that happens over time. You don't just let a partner try penetration with a finger then try intercourse three minutes later, which is not enough time to prepare you for sex physically. Each person is different in their need for time and preparation for sexual intercourse. However, as an estimate, ideally, you may want to try vaginal insertion at least 6 or 7 times with a finger over at least a few days prior to attempting intercourse. Next, try using two fingers, going through the same process. After this period of preparation, you may be ready for sexual intercourse with a penis.

Virgin sex is a process, not an event.

For "Lisa," whose story appeared earlier in this chapter, sex was a pleasurable experience, but full penetration with a penis took place over several days, with full sexual thrusting taking two months. Take your time in preparing to lose your virginity, and even in having first sexual experiences. Even if it's been a while since you've had intercourse, your vagina needs to be prepared for sexual penetration for you to be ready for full sexual action, and to have fun! After exploring sexual penetration with fingers, if you are emotionally ready, you will probably be physically ready for sexual intercourse with a penis. Your vagina has a thin layer of skin, called your hymen, which is at the entrance of your vagina. Your hymen needs to be gently opened. Often, by the time a woman has intercourse, her hymen is already opened and there isn't any pain. With the process of preparing your vagina with the insertion and movement of fingers, it is likely that the opening of the vagina has been expanded and the skin of the hymen is already gone. If your hymen is still in place or if it's unusually thick, there may be some bleeding and slight discomfort in opening it to allow sexual intercourse. For this reason, the insertion of the penis needs to take place very slowly to open the hymen, which may require a gentle push. When this is forced and done incorrectly, the hymen skin may tear or burst open, which is why bad sex is called "popping the cherry."

Prior to entering your vagina, his penis needs to be lubricated: with the wetness from the lubricant on a condom, by moving the head of his penis across the inner lips of your naturally moistened vulva, or using saliva, so that he can slide easily into your vagina. It is often helpful if you hold his penis with your hand and guide it slowly to the opening of your vagina, although he may also be able to find the opening. At first, put just the head of his penis inside you. If this causes no discomfort, continue penetration as far as your vagina will allow without pain. If full penetration is not possible, practice penetration over a few days, or over a longer period of time if necessary, until his penis can comfortably fit inside of your vagina. Make sure that your vagina is always lubricated and moist for comfortable penetration. If necessary, alternate between penetration on one day with his penis and the next with his finger to stretch out your vagina and prepare for sex. Also, don't limit your love-making to intercourse: continue kissing, touching, looking into each other's eyes and feeling other parts of each other's bodies. For one thing, you want to stay excited, but you also want to share affection and love. Once full penetration is possible, begin to slowly allow him to move his penis in and out of your vagina without his penis completely leaving your vagina. Take your time with increasing the speed and depth of thrusting. Most guys will be so excited that they will want to "go for it" and get into full thrusting, driving their penis fast and hard inside of you, until they come. Some guys have the idea that the harder they push and deeper they go the more you will like it. This may be true for you later on, but at first, you need to set the pace for sexual intercourse. You can do this by moving and positioning your hips, holding onto to his hips and using your hands to move him faster or slower, or by telling him to speed up or slow down.

If this is an early sexual experience for your boyfriend, he may have difficulty controlling his orgasm or ejaculation. Many young men get easily excited with first sexual experiences, and they may come very quickly, sometimes even before sexual penetration happens. This is called "premature ejaculation," and it's a common experience for young men, but it happens with more experienced men, too. This is usually embarrassing for guys, and it can be an uncomfortable situation for both of you, but it doesn't have to be! Be understanding and patient with your boyfriend, reassuring him that you know it's a very normal and it happens. The great thing about young guys is that if you just wait several minutes, he will be able to get another erection, and you can try again later. You can go back to talking and listening, or touching and feeling, to continue to express loving feelings and share sexual touch in other ways.

At any time that you feel uncomfortable or experience pain, emotionally or physically, whether it is your first time or the 50th time, ask your partner to stop or slow down. Go back to the basics: talking and listening. If things go "wrong" and nothing seems to be clicking together once in a while, don't worry about it and don't blame each other. Just as with anything in life, timing can be off, unpredictable events interrupt you, and you can change your mood. Use your sexual communication skills to talk about how you feel, especially if you ever feel pain, and tell your partner what you want to do differently. Say STOP if you want to stop, even if you're in the middle of a heated sexual moment. It's OK! Stop if you just aren't feeling any sexual excitement in one situation.

Sometimes, you will feel sexually aroused from sexual touch and sexual intercourse, and the next time you may do exactly the same things on a different day, but you won't feel the same. If sexual intercourse isn't working for you or doesn't feel good, go back to other kinds of sexual touch that feel pleasurable to you, or wait until another day, when you are in a different mood. Women feel differently sexually depending on how they feel emotionally toward their partner, different hormonal times in their menstrual cycles, stress, and how they feel emotionally and physically that day. Be flexible as a couple of what you choose to experience on any given day, but remember to always share pleasure and never pain. The important thing to remember is that sex is about sharing love, and if you start and continue with talking and listening, you can work out the very normal day to day, week to week changes that occur in sexual relationships.

> If you and your partner work together to make virgin sex right, sex can be a lifelong pleasure, filled with intimacy and love.

## WHAT TEENS THINK ABOUT AFTER SEX

OK, now you have thought about everything you think you need to consider before making a decision about having sex. Now what do you do after sex, to make sure everything is emotionally right for you and your partner? After making love for the first time, most girls and guys don't know the right things to say or do. They are not sure what to say when it comes to sharing emotional or physical feelings. Virgin sex is a sharing of a very special part of your being for the first time in your life. Many people experience a very deep emotional and physical closeness for the very first time in their lives. Yet, some people, especially those who don't have an emotional connection with their partner, don't feel much different and they wonder, "What's the big deal?" For almost all young men and women, this is a new kind of closeness that they have never experienced before, and they simply don't know what to do or say because they have never been in this situation. Here are guidelines to starting things off right.

> The truth is: Sexual closeness is different than almost anything you will experience in your life. It will change your relationship with your partner and your relationship with yourself forever.

# Dr. Darcy's After Sex Guide

- Right after sex, talk to him about how you feel and what you thought about what you experienced.

- Right after sex, lie together and hold each other. Don't get scared and just run off.

- Guys really want to know if they "performed" OK (great is even better) or if their penises were big enough. These are guy's two biggest insecurities. Reassure them. Also, tell him if you enjoyed yourself and if you had sexual pleasure.

- Reassure him that you are probably not pregnant because you (and this better be the case) have taken precautions against pregnancy.

- Talk to him and keep the lines of communication open.

- Do talk to your best friend, if you have one, and if you ABSOLUTELY trust her or him to keep this news private. You do not want anyone to start spreading rumors about you.

- Don't put the expectation on yourself that you have to have sex again, unless you want to.

- Especially with same sex relationships with girls: Remind her that this was private . . . just between you two. No one wants someone else to decide when they should come out.

Joyful sexual expression is the result of two people exploring sex together, with both of them using their own sexual voice in one act of harmonious love.

# Virgin Sex Reminders

- A woman needs to have emotional sexual desire first, then arousal, then sexual play before she makes a decision about sexual penetration.

- Intercourse is reserved only for a moment in time when both partners first and foremost feel completely comfortable with the sexual pleasuring.

- Sexual intercourse is a process, not an event—that often requires several days of preparation in order to avoid physical pain the first time.

- When a girl says no or stop, the guy has to stop regardless of the stage of sexual play or this is rape.

# ten

# WHAT EVERY GIRL NEEDS TO KNOW ABOUT RAPE AND SEXUAL ABUSE

All girls must be knowledgeable about rape and sexual abuse. Most girls will find reading this chapter difficult, but it is important to understand. Some people think rape and sexual abuse hardly ever happen. This is not true. One in four girls in America is sexually abused before she is 18. That means that you have a 25% chance of being sexually abused, if it hasn't already happened, before you are 18. Some statistics show that 1 in 4 women are date raped or "acquaintance raped" in college. Looking at it this way, sexual abuse and rape are common experiences in America. If you are already a victim of sexual abuse or rape, this chapter may contain some stories or information that remind you of your experiences and it may be difficult to read. If you have never experienced sexual abuse or rape, this chapter may help prevent you from becoming another abused person.

This chapter is written to help young women understand what sexual abuse is, what rape is, and how you can identify it, and hopefully, prevent it. I wish NO ONE ever had to experience sexual trauma, but the facts are the facts. Such trauma can have devastating effects on a girl's sexual self, self-esteem, view of sex in general, mental health, and future sexual attitudes and experiences. Trauma particularly affects a woman's trust in men, and in seeing the world as a safe place in general.

All young women need to be aware of the possible ways that sex can be abusive, how to avoid such abuse, and what to do if it happens to you or a friend. Sexual abuse has many definitions, so these are summarized here for you. A few women who have experienced sexual abuse courageously share their stories in this chapter and tell how sexual abuse or rape happened and how it affected them, sexually and emotionally.

WARNING TO TEENS AND THEIR PARENTS: This chapter contains sexually detailed information about sexual abuse, rape, and young women's real stories of their experiences with sexual trauma or difficult sexual experiences. While efforts have been made to prevent presenting this information in a sexually explicit manner, some of the content may be shocking to young teenagers. While many teenagers may benefit from understanding sexual abuse and rape, younger teens may choose not to read the stories in this section. After the section on "Common Types of Molestation," a young teen might want to skip to the section on "What are the Causes of Rape?"

## COMMON TYPES OF SEXUAL ABUSE

**Exhibitionism or Exposure:** Displaying of the naked body or parts of the naked body in an effort to shock, intimidate, or sexually arouse a victim.

**Molestation:** Sexual abuse involving sexual stimulation to body and genital areas, usually by touch, but also including penis to vagina or mouth. It can happen at any age and by a perpetrator of any age.

**Child Sexual Abuse:** Sexual abuse of children by adults or by older children or peers who dominate and control through sexual activity. Older boys may make girls undress and then touch them genitally, for example. Childhood sexual abuse can be committed by a stranger, but most often it is done by adults or older children in trusted care-taking roles. A rule of thumb for "normal sexual exploration" by children with children is an age difference of no more than 3 years, and includes undressing, nudity, hugging and kissing, but not sexual touch.

**Incest:** Incest is the most common form of child sexual abuse. Incest is sexual abuse of children by other family members, including mothers or fathers, sisters and brothers, stepparents, aunts, uncles, cousins, and grandparents.

**Date or Acquaintance Rape:** Sexual abuse and sexual behavior for which there is no verbal or nonverbal permission. This type of rape may be sexual assault, but it is not necessarily violent. Date rape is committed by someone known to the victim, often a peer in a trusted social relationship.

**Stranger Rape:** Violence, anger, and power expressed sexually in an attack on a victim. It may involve penetration of body openings (mouth, anus, vagina), but it does not have to. Stranger rape is a sexual attack committed by someone unknown to the victim.

**Marital Rape:** Rape of a spouse or marital partner.

**Sexual Assault:** A physical attack to a victim's sexual body parts, often involving force or violence. This term can cover a wide rage of activities and can include the rape of boys and men.

**Voyeurism:** An invasion of a victim's privacy either secretively or openly with the intent of gaining sexual gratification. Commonly, this can mean watching someone having sexual relations, watching someone dress, or just watching someone for sexual gratification, such as a man in a truck stalking a girl in a car while she is riding down the highway with a short skirt on. This person can also be called a "peeping Tom."

**Obscene Phone Calls:** An invasion of a victim's privacy with sexually suggestive messages over the telephone in an effort to shock, intimidate, or sexually arouse a victim. Often the offender will be doing this for sexual excitement and may be masturbating.

**Statutory Rape:** If you are younger than a certain age, having sex is child sexual abuse, even if you say "yes." If you are younger than the "age of consent," anyone having sex with you is committing statutory rape. "Statutory" means it is a crime because of your status, the "status" in this case being a minor who is not the age of consent. The age of consent is how old a child must be to legally say it is OK to have sexual touch or sexual intercourse, or else it is legally considered sexual assault or molestation or rape. The idea is that young people could be coerced into sex, which means that they are not yet ready to make this decision based on their own conditions for sex and so they might be having sex because they were talked into it. See Chapter 4 on "The Legal Bottom Line" on sex.

**Sadistic Sexual Abuse:** Sadistic means cruel or vicious. Sexual abuse in which the offender incites or tries to incite reactions of dread, horror, or pain in the victim, often increasing the offender's sexual arousal during the abuse, is sadistic sexual abuse. This may involve use of physical restraint, religious types of rituals, multiple perpetrators, animals, and torture.

**Sexual Exploitation:** Using a person as a thing, not as a real person, or "objectifying" or using a victim in sexual activity or photographic imagery to gain money or sexual gratification.

**Sexual Harassment:** Generally, sexual harassment happens in a school or workplace, where a person uses his or her power or status to intimidate or control a victim, perhaps requiring sexual involvement. One type of sexual harassment may be expressed as excessive sexual flirtatiousness, and/or requests for sexual favors to obtain something from the abused, such as undressing or having sex for a good grade in a class. The other type of sexual harassment involves creating a "sexually hostile" environment, such as continually making degrading comments about women, displaying explicit sexual pictures, or telling dirty sex jokes.

**Gender Attack:** An exposure to actions that demean the sexual gender of a victim, often with sexual overtones, such as cross-dressing a child or verbally denigrating a victim's gender.

**Gay Bashing:** Verbal or physical attacks directed against a victim's perceived homosexual orientation.

**Sexual Violence:** Acts of violence involving or harming or violating the sexual parts of the victim's body.

## THE INTERNET: A CAUTIONARY TALE

Instant messaging is the most popular way to socialize through the Internet. In the 1950's it was the "soda shop," where our grandparents went to drink cherry cokes and hang out with friends. In the 70's, it was the telephone. Having your own "teen phone," to talk on for 2 or 3 hours a day was the way 14 year olds "got together." Now, teens use the Internet and chat online, whether on AOL or AIM, to socialize.

Teens can talk to teens from their local hometown to Singapore to anywhere in the world on the Internet. As many as 80% of teens are online, with many of them using instant messaging to reach out to friends or get to know new friends they might meet in chatrooms. Instant messaging or "IMing" as a way to socialize is a fun, quick, and easy way to stay in touch with friends. Having four screens going at a time and typing quickly is a way to keep your social life moving fast.

Most of the time, it is a safe and fun way to "get together." Yet, the amazing statistic is that 15% (FIFTEEN percent) of teens actually meet people they meet online LIVE and in person (http://ncecc.ca/enviroscan_2005_e.html, 2006). Often these meetings are private, secretive, without parental knowledge or consent, with teens meeting strangers they have only 'met' online.

Kids are taught, "Don't talk to strangers," from the time they can understand language. Yet, as teens, millions of people are meeting strangers everyday on the Internet, and thousands of teens are meeting strangers in person every year. Strange, isn't it? You know not to talk to strangers, yet, it has become commonplace to talk to people you don't really know online every day! Making the leap from the anonymous contact of the world wide web and Internet chatting to meeting a person live can seem very different than the warnings we were taught as children, to stay away from strangers. After "talking" or chatting online, in a very short period of time, people can begin to feel very close, and experience feelings as deeply as if they were meeting in person. In fact, some people report feeling they have fallen in love with someone they have never even met in person, because the feelings of emotional connection from communicating online were so strong. So, the leap from being anonymous to meeting what seems to be a new, very best friend, doesn't seem like it is in the same category of meeting a stranger. Yet, in fact, you are meeting a stranger and it is very dangerous!

Meeting a stranger you have 'met' online is very risky behavior.

People can pretend to be anyone they want to be online. A 50 year old, hairy, wrinkled old man, who is attracted to children can pretend to be hot 16 year old guy (or girl) who loves the same music as you do. Sex offenders "target and groom" intended victims of child sexual abuse. Child sexual predators use teenage chatrooms to get individual email addresses, then use instant messaging to have "relationships," then prey on teens like an animal preys on another animal. Many teenagers have met in person "new friends" they have met online, and some of them have been sexually assaulted and even murdered. Teenagers are at great risk for becoming victims of child abuse, pornography, or even human trafficking (prostitution), when they meet strangers they have met online on the Internet.

## Dos and Don'ts of the Internet

- Do not use an Internet name that has personal information, such as the name of your high school, town, or sport, e.g. "WashingtonHighCheerleader2010!"
- Never give out your phone number.
- Never give out your home town or address information.
- Do not tell your real name, especially your last name. Always use a nickname that your real friends already know.
- If you begin to feel uncomfortable when talking and meeting people online, leave the site and turn off your computer immediately.
- Do tell someone if someone starts asking really personal or inappropriate and/or sexual questions. If someone starts asking you a lot of personal questions, report them to https://web.cybertip.org/cyberTipII.html.
- Do not meet anyone you meet online.
- If you feel you must meet someone, always tell a parent, meet in a public place, and go with someone while having your own transportation to come and leave.

- Remember that if you call someone, they can get your phone number from their cell phone or they can get call *69 to get your number. If you ever make a phone call, don't call a cell phone number, or dial *67 first to block your phone number. If someone has your phone number, they can get your home address!

- A legitimate person will have no problems with your parents knowing you are meeting them.

- A real friend will not require you to keep their friendship or meeting secret.

## TYPES OF CHILD SEXUAL ABUSE

Wendy Maltz (1991), an author and expert on sexual abuse, writes:

> "Sexual abuse occurs whenever one person dominates and exploits another by means of sexual activity or suggestion. Sexual feelings and behavior that are used to degrade, humiliate, control, hurt, or otherwise misuse another person are sexually abusive. Coercion or betrayal often plays into sexual abuse. The abuse can take a direct, painful and obvious course, such as in stranger rape. Or abuse can be indirect, perhaps even subtle, such as when a victim is gently fondled by an offender who professes love." (Pg. 31).

### Child Sexual Abuse—Logan's Story

Logan came from an upper middle class family, which looked, on the outside like "the perfect family." However, Logan was sexually molested beginning at the age of 3. She was touched on the genitals by her own father, on many occasions, and over several years, until her parents divorced. Logan's abuse was emotional, as well as sexual, because she felt betrayed by her father, who was supposed to love and protect her. Also, her father would take her out to the bar with him, have her dressed up cute and perfect, and act like they were on a "date" together until she was around 12.

Logan's mother was addicted to pills and alcohol and didn't really notice anything much going on with Logan. She did take good care of Logan in many ways. Logan had the finest of clothes, was clean, well educated, and well fed. To anyone outside of the family, Logan looked like a very normal girl.

Her mother remarried when Logan was 13. After the marriage, her stepfather started to sexually abuse her. He touched her breasts and would insist, even at that age, to have her sit on his lap. He would touch her vulva and penetrate her vagina with his finger. His penis would get erect when she sat on his lap and she would feel it. He'd rock her back and forth and have an orgasm when he was touching her. Logan told her mother what was happening, but her mother was in complete denial about the situation and told Logan, "He's only showing you that he loves you." Logan didn't know any better.

Logan's sexual abuse took place in the early 1960s, and at the time people generally didn't believe that sexual abuse happened and they certainly didn't talk about it when it did. Logan just thought that sexual play happened in all families. She didn't really know that other people DIDN'T do it, because no one talked about it. Basically, from her early sexual experiences, she learned that "SEX is LOVE." Yet, she felt that sex was "yucky" and "gross" and she didn't want to have anything to do with it.

Logan went to college "a virgin" because she was taught by her mother and the church not to have sex until she got married [ironic, isn't it?]. Logan dated some guys in high school, and she was very pretty, but she didn't want to have anything to do with sex. Sadly, when Logan was in college at 19, she was walking home at night from work and she was brutally raped. She was physically beaten, bruised, scarred, and left for dead in an alley. At that point, she decided she hated sex and she didn't trust men or the world.

Logan had her first welcomed, voluntary, and consensual sexual relationship at 21. She fell in love with a man she thought she would marry and she wanted to make love with him. Not surprisingly, Logan hated sex: it hurt, it made her feel angry, and she felt it was very unpleasant overall. She believes now that she just had so many unpleasant memories associated with sex that she couldn't enjoy it. It wasn't the guy: it was her.

Logan married in her early 20s, choosing an emotionally distant and mentally abusive man to marry. She didn't have very good ideas about what a good man or husband should be like. After many unhappy years, she got divorced. It was then that she started therapy to try to heal her wounds from childhood as well as from her bad marriage.

At age 40, Logan finally met and dated a guy several years younger than she was who was a tender, loving and patient man named "Blease." It took her 40 years, 37 years after her first abusive experiences with sex, to enjoy sex. Although it started slowly, Blease was a safe, trusting, and patient sexual partner who never pressured or pushed himself on Logan. She feels like she had her sexual birth at 40 years old.

Nowadays, the public is much more aware of the reality of sexual abuse and there are serious criminal laws against people who commit sexual crimes. If you are like most girls and guys, your parents and/or schools have taught you, from a very young age, that no one is allowed to touch your "private parts," and you should tell someone if it happens. However, sexual abuse remains frighteningly common, and I have young girls or young women come forward to tell me about sexual abuse every month. It still happens. Girls still do not want to tell anyone about sexual abuse, especially if the abuser is a parent, a stepparent, or a family friend: girls are afraid no one will believe them and they don't want to get anyone in trouble. It is a reality that child molesters and rapists can be put in prison and this will cause many problems and/or may break up a family. No one wants their dad or uncle to go to jail! Also, many young girls still blame themselves for sexual abuse, especially if they will get into trouble for being in a certain situation, like being at friend's house when the parents weren't home.

Remember, it is NEVER a young girl's fault if she is sexually abused, under ANY circumstances. Adults know that it is WRONG and ILLEGAL to have sex with a girl or boy who is under 18 or the age of consent (see "statutory rape"). In fact, adults who abuse children often use embarrassment, guilt, and blame as a weapon to keep victims silent. Or sex offenders make threats against a child or their family, such as, "I'll tell everyone that you are a little whore and a liar," or "I'll get your sister next or hurt your family if you ever tell anyone." These threats feel very real, but the real threat is that child sexual abusers fear they will get in trouble. THERE IS PROTECTION and treatment for victims of sexual abuse.

## Sexual Exposure—Jenna's Story

Jenna experienced "exposure" when she was about 7 years old. She lived in a nice subdivision on Long Island, New York, and she spent a lot of time playing outdoors. One day, there was an older kid riding around the neighborhood on his bike whom she had never seen before. He was around 13 or 14. A couple of times, he lifted up his long t-shirt revealing nothing underneath. He wore no shorts and no underwear, showing his privates in plain view in the daylight.

Mostly, Jenna was grossed out at the sight of this naked kid on his bike. He was kind of fat and his stomach hung disgustingly over his crotch, but not far enough to cover his genitals. Jenna never told her parents, because she really didn't know how bad it was that this fat, weird looking teenage boy exposed himself. Also, Jenna figured her parents would make her stay inside if she told them about him and she didn't want to be stuck inside the house all day. It was summer and she wanted to be free to be outside and play.

At first, Jenna was not sure if anyone else in her family saw this, as she had two older brothers, but she later heard about some boy getting into trouble for riding around and "exposing himself" in public. She figured it must have been that kid, but Jenna never said a word. It was, literally, her first exposure to sexual abuse. All she knew was that it was "gross."

As a result, as a young woman, Jenna didn't particularly look forward to seeing a naked man. Later in life, she finally realized that this incident was probably why she avoided seeing men naked.

243

Exposure can have quite a lot of different effects on girls and women. Feelings can vary from giggles to horror to fear for one's life. What is important is that you tell someone if this ever happens to you. If you think about it a lot or have nightmares, talk to a parent or counselor, or even your sister, brother, cousin or friend. Having someone jump right across your "sexual boundaries" can be traumatic and is sexual abuse. Exposure can be a shock to you that can change your feelings about sex in general, and it can affect special parts of sex in the future.

## Sexual Molestation

Being molested means exactly what the word says. Molested means being BOTHERED. Sexual molestation means being bothered and sexually touched, without your permission, but without vaginal or anal intercourse. Generally, molestation refers to touching or fondling of the breasts or genitals with the hands or a rubbing against someone with their sexual parts. One example is being on a bus or subway and having a man rub his hard penis or erection against you, but molestation can also be touching or fondling of the breasts, buttocks, or genitals. Molestation includes a child sitting on the lap of a man when he has an erection and is making contact of his penis with the child, either just sitting there or making rubbing or rocking motions. In almost all cases, molestation does not refer to parents giving spankings to a child for disciplinarian purposes. Molestation does include when someone might slip their hand across your buttocks, across your chest, or down your pants to touch your genitals, and you know it was not an "accident." In most cases, a sexual offender is someone you know, like a family friend, neighbor, coach, or even a brother or his friend.

All of these behaviors are wrong when they are not welcomed, when you are not old enough for sex, or they are not "consensual." "Consensual" means that you say "yes" and give permission for someone to touch you. Generally, molestation refers to someone touching you who is in a position of authority or power over you, such as a teacher, a coach, your mother's boyfriend, or a neighbor, WHETHER YOU SAY YES, if you are not the age of "consent," OR YOU SAY NO OR YOU ARE SILENT.

> Even if you "agree," an adult has no right to touch you on the breasts, buttocks, or genitals, no matter what, if you are not the age of consent.

At a certain age, you are considered old enough to give consent for sexual touch or sexual intercourse. Having your boyfriend, as long as he is also under 18, touch your breast, buttocks, or genitals is not sexual abuse if you say it is OK. If you say stop and he doesn't stop, even if his hand is down your pants and outside your vagina at the time but you changed your mind, he needs to stop. Move his hand, tell him to stop and respect your verbal wishes, statements, or demands or it is sexual abuse.

Who cares if they like you or not?

You have to like you. . . . today and tomorrow and the rest of your life.

In reality, very few people make a report to the police about molestation. Most people don't consider it to be "rape." Therefore, what are the police going to do about it? Besides, who would believe you? Besides, how embarrassing to tell someone about it! Besides, how would you prove it anyway . . . it is just your word against theirs!

Sexual molestation IS A CRIME as well as being unwanted touch. Yes, it is not considered as serious a crime as rape, but it is against the law. It is just considered a different "degree" or type of sexual assault. But, for some girls, sexual molestation is just as devastating as actually being raped. IT COUNTS. IT WEAKENS YOUR TRUST FOR THE WORLD AND FOR MEN. Remember this: some perverted people who molest people "only molest" them because they have gotten away with it, often or many times. Sometimes reporting this crime establishes a beginning of a crime record so that if it happens again the police can get a profile of the person and gather evidence. You could help some other girl (or guy) in the future. IT IS A BIG DEAL. It is your body and you have a right not to be touched if it is unwanted or you are underage.

245

## Examples of Molestation

*Example #1: What about when a doctor is examining and touches you, especially for a gynecological exam?*

It is OK for a doctor to examine and touch you when medically necessary; however, in most states, when a doctor is giving a pelvic exam, a female nurse is required to be present to prevent anything other than a proper exam. You can also have a friend, a relative, or your parent present. They don't have to watch an exam. It's OK for them to just be there, possibly from a "shoulder" view with pelvic exams, to make you feel more comfortable. Even when you are uncomfortable when a doctor is touching your body or even the inside of your body, like with a rectal or vaginal exam, this is not sexual molestation or sexual abuse, even when it may not feel right. You will have to work on getting comfortable with medical sexual contact, so you can take care of your physical health. In rare cases, a medical professional may "go too far" with sexual touch, and in these cases their touching is sexual molestation. This is why a nurse is present to monitor a pelvic exam in most states in the US.

246

*Example #2: What about when your younger brother pulls your bathing suit or your halter top up or down?*

It isn't uncommon in families for a younger (or older) brother to think it's funny to grab at your clothes and make you feel embarrassed in public, nor is it unusual that he might like to steal a peek. Most of the time, this is not considered ABUSE, but such behavior is inappropriate. This is being BOTHERED. Your parent or parents need to be told what happened and step in to correct the situation. Your brother needs to understand what he is doing is hurting you and is wrong. He also needs to have some kind of consequences or punishment, so he will think first before doing it again. Repeated behavior of this sort, despite consequences, can be a sign of more serious problems.

*Example #3: What do you do when you're making out and he is going faster and farther than you want to go?*

Often guys will start exploring your body with their hands, almost before you can speak up or move your hand to stop them. If you don't want the touch, then you have to be very direct with guys. Guys don't know what it is like to be a girl and what it is like to have a girl's body: they usually think its great when you grab them. They may be very curious, in love with you, or just horny, but make sure you stay in control with your voice and your body.

This is a COMMON situation. Even if a guy likes you, some guys forget to think about who you are and your values and think about their own sex drive. Some guys are jerks and are only interested in getting "as far as they can get" to experience what a girl's body feels like. If things are moving too fast or going too far, gently pushing his hand away and softly saying, "Uh, I don't know about this" is not going to control the situation. You have to be FIRM AND DIRECT. A man's hands and bodies are usually stronger than those of a girl. The firm, quick movements they make to your crotch or under your shirt are with strength. Use the strength of your voice and also use your strength in your own hands to FIRMLY move their hands or legs or any other body parts away from you if you are not comfortable with what is happening.

If a guy doesn't listen to your voice or body gestures, stand up! Move! Walk away! Get out of the car! Get out of the room! Get out of the house! Go home! If this does not work . . . then scream and yell at him to leave you alone!

At this point, it doesn't matter what he wants . . . all that matters is how you feel and what you need to do to feel comfortable and to be safe. Often guys have two different parts in their mind, like the little angel or devil you see in cartoons sitting above each shoulder. The angel says to you, "I really care about you and your feelings, and I want to listen to you." The devil says, "I'm sexually excited and want to get as far as I can get sexually." While it is wrong, sometimes guys can get sexually carried away in sexual situations from their excitement, and in such cases they listen to the "devil" in them. This is one reason girls need to be cautious about making decisions about how far they want to go with a guy and talk about it with him before getting alone with him in a potentially sexual situation. Nevertheless, a guy is responsible for his own behavior and listening to you, too. If a guy doesn't listen to you and doesn't stop when you tell him to, it is called sexual molestation if he touches you sexually without your permission and it's against the law.

## Incest—Danielle's Story

Danielle was a client's daughter. She was anally raped, or sodomized, by her cousin when she was about 5 years old. That means this guy put his penis into her anus. It happened to her twice. Danielle never told anyone until she was 15, except her brother. Her brother is two years older than she is and they were close friends. He was a really sweet boy, and it was a godsend that at least she had someone with whom to share her secret.

She never told anyone because her sexual abuser was her 12-year-old cousin. When it happened, she didn't even know what it was, except that it hurt really badly. After the second time, she just avoided ever being in the same room with him and stayed very close to her mom or her older, bigger brother when her cousin came around. Danielle never told her mom because she figured that her mom would tell her dad. Danielle had been told by both of her parents to never let anyone touch her private parts. She was told from about the age of 3 that her privates were PRIVATE and no one else could touch them. Her father was a loving protective father, but he also had a temper. He had said to his children on more than one occasion "if anyone ever messed with one of you kids, I'd kill him." Her daddy owned a couple of guns and knew how to use them. Danielle and her brother believed their dad, and while they appreciated his fatherly love and protection for them, they didn't dare tell him because they didn't want to see their cousin dead. They also didn't want to see their Aunt's heart broken to hear that her child was a sexual perpetrator. Poor Danielle didn't want to break up her Aunt's family, make her grandma feel bad, and she didn't want to see her daddy go to jail for killing someone.

So, Danielle kept silent for ten years. It was when she was in high school that she broke her silence to her mother. Her mother believed her and brought her to a counselor to talk about it. This was after the cousin had recently died in a car accident, so Danielle felt she could safely break her silence without the police being involved.

The effect of sexual abuse and silence on Danielle was very bad. Ever since she was in first grade, she didn't want to dress like a "pretty girl" anymore. In fact, she dressed more like a boy: big t-shirts and baggy jeans were her style. She didn't want any guys to look at her or touch her sexually. She even got teased at school for being a "dyke," that is, she was accused of being gay, even though Danielle knew she wasn't. She just didn't want any guys looking at her or touching her. By the time she got to high school, she had had her share of crushes on guys but she had never acted on them because she didn't trust boys.

Danielle's therapy was about reclaiming her femininity and uncovering her strikingly good looks, as well as about developing friendships with guys. For her, the "first time" was unwelcome and painful. She had to learn how to be a girl and a sexual person all over again. In her senior year in high school, Danielle had her first boyfriend and she fell totally "in love." With guidance from her mom and therapy, she had a very positive first sexual experience.

Incest is particularly devastating, because it not only involves sexual betrayal but emotional betrayal as well. It will shake your world to not be able to trust someone who is supposed to be your loving family member. Almost all people who have experienced incest need professional help to overcome this trauma and violation in order to truly become a sexual assault "survivor."

A common question for incest and sexual assault survivors is: "If I was raped, am I still a virgin?" Technically, a girl is not a virgin when her hymen has been torn by penetration with a penis, although many girls wonder about their virginity. Almost all sexual abuse survivors consider themselves to be "virgins" until they have consensual sex, or when they say "yes" to sex. Some girls call this their "real virginity," or "secondary virginity."

## TYPES OF RAPE

### Stranger Rape

Rape by a stranger is what most people think about when they hear about rape. People think of a stranger coming out of the bushes, in the dark, jumping on someone, and forcing them to have sex. Actually, stranger rape is much less common than incest and acquaintance rape, but it does happen. Every young woman should know about and protect themselves against high-risk situations that can hurt them. Of course, there is no fool-proof method of self-protection from rape by a stranger, but the following advice should be heeded.

## Avoiding Stranger Rape

- Do not walk home by yourself in the dark.
- Be careful of walking near bushes.
- Do not look like a victim: don't act confused or unaware of your surroundings.
- Don't give out your last name or address at parties or bars. If strongly pressured, make up a name.
- Avoid malls, grocery store parking lots, and parking garages at night.

- Beware of faked car accidents, where someone will hit your car and when you stop, rob or rape you.
- Beware of set-up situations at malls, where a man will ask you to go to the parking lot to help with a screaming baby, a sick mother, broken down car, etc.
- Have good locks on your home or apartment, especially a dead bolt, and use them every day.
- Do not give out your name, number or address or password on the Internet.
- Learn basic self-defense techniques.
- Do not list your full first name in the telephone directory: it shows you're a single woman.
- Some young women feel more comfortable getting a dog if they live alone.

## Acquaintance and Date Rape

Acquaintance rape is forced, unwanted sexual intercourse by a person the victim knows. Date rape is forced, unwanted sex with someone the victim is dating. Both types of rape are a violation of your body and your trust and can be a violation by someone you have just met or dated a few times, or even with just a friend or casual acquaintance. Research estimates that 90% of rapes are never reported and 60% of victims know their rapists. But with teenage victims of such assaults, it is estimated that 92% know the sexual perpetrator (womensissues. about.com/od/rapecrisis/a/rapestats.htm). One website reports that 28% of women are raped by their boyfriends and a rape occurs every 2 minutes in the United States. Very interestingly, however, only 57% of women who have been raped called the incident "rape." Most likely it's because they knew the rapist and, in part, blamed themselves for the incident, questioning what really happened.

You can look for the early warning signs of rape, and if you know how to react to them you can take steps to avoid it. You can not avoid all rape situations, but you can do your best to avoid some of them, if you learn from what you are about to read and act carefully. Only twenty years ago, no one ever heard of, or at least talked about, date rape. Forty years ago, girls had to have "chaperones" or supervision on dates. Since that practice stopped, my guess is that there has been a huge increase of acquaintance or date rape. What we do know is that about 1 in 4 college women are victims of date rape. Since young women aren't going to want to start being "chaperoned" on dates, when you are finally allowed to be alone with a guy at 15 or 16, you need to start thinking and acting in a self-protective way to avoid being raped.

## Dee's Story

Dee was date raped when she was 18 and a sophomore (in her 2nd year) in college. Dave was a guy who lived in her college dorm. The college had "coed" dorms, which meant guys and girls lived in the same building. Dave lived on a different floor than Dee. He had gone to the same high school as Dee, although he was a year or two ahead of her in school. He was on the baseball team at school, so he was an athlete like she was (she played softball) so they had a lot in common. Dee had frequently been on Dave's floor to visit male friends who were also on the baseball team. Dee had felt very comfortable on the men's floor, as she had had many male friends, some who were somewhat protective of the women on the softball team, and no guys had EVER been sexually inappropriate in the year and a half that she was at college or living in the dormitory. Over the previous month, Dee had begun to visit Dave and his roommate in their dorm room on several brief occasions. Generally, there were one or more other guys or girls around: everyone was just hanging out, talking, or listening to music. The atmosphere was casual and friendly.

Dave, Dee, and several other people had had a few beers that night and it got late. The group of friends thinned out and those who remained wanted to go to sleep, so they went back to their dorm rooms, leaving just Dave and Dee in his room. Since there wasn't much to do, Dee invited Dave up to her room to watch TV because he had no TV in his room. Her dorm room was set up comfortably with a couch and television, and the beds were in an overhead "loft" so the dorm room had a living room atmosphere that was relaxed and comfortable. Dee's roommate was gone for the night. After the TV show they were watching ended, Dee asked Dave to leave. That's when the trouble started.

Dave refused to leave. He said he was tired and just wanted to sleep on the large couch, which folded into a bed like a futon. Dee said no. She asked him repeatedly to leave. He refused. She went to the door to leave herself and Dave blocked the door and bolted it from the inside. Dave was pretty drunk and Dee thought he was acting irrationally. She felt powerless. She was afraid he was going to hurt her seriously or even kill her. He strongly refused to leave and wouldn't let her leave either, stating that he wanted to sleep in her room overnight. Feeling helpless, Dee suggested he just go to sleep on the sofa bed. Dee hoped he would sleep off his drunkenness and act normal in the morning.

In the middle of the night, Dee awoke to Dave climbing on top of her, holding her arms down and starting to have sex with her. All she could get out of her mouth was, "What are you doing?" The next thing she knew he was pulling down his pants, lifting up her skirt and forcing his penis inside her vagina. She struggled a little, but she was half asleep, half drunk, and felt defenseless. Most importantly, she was afraid for her life. She felt that if she struggled anymore he might just hurt her. So, she pretended to fall back asleep and he "finished" quickly. He fell asleep, then woke up early in the morning and left her room.

What Every Girl Needs to Know About Rape and Sexual Abuse

Dee woke up early in the morning, stone-cold sober, and thought over what had happened. She blamed herself for his having sexual intercourse with her, because she had invited him into her room, she had been flirtatious with him, she had been drinking, and she thought she "let" him sleep in her room that night.

Dee did not call what happened rape for a long time.

Dee blamed herself for being "so stupid" and not firmly and directly telling him "NO!" when he was forcing himself on top of her in the middle of the night. She blamed herself for what happened because she didn't start screaming and yelling for help. The next day, Dave came back to her dorm room and apologized. He begged her not to tell anyone and he promised that it would never happen again. He said he was very sorry.

Dee never reported it to the police. She regrets not reporting it to the police to this day. She never reported it because she did not want to have everyone in the small school to know what happened. Dee blamed herself for the fact that he had sex with her. She felt she was responsible for being raped because she let Dave into her room and she did not REALLY say NO. Also, Dee did not want to be stared at and judged by everyone in the school. Dee had known one other girl at school who was raped and everyone talked so much about her that the girl left school. Dee was attending college on a scholarship; she desperately wanted to get her education and she didn't feel that leaving school was an option for her. Most importantly, Dee did not feel the police would believe her and it was just her word against Dave's.

Dave was from a popular family. His father was well known in their hometown and they were well liked. Basically, the circumstances of the assault came down to Dee's word against his, and she was a "nobody." Dee didn't even know about "rape tests" or "sperm collection tests" that might have helped her case. Dee also did not want her parents to know, because she felt they would blame her, too. Also, she didn't want her whole family to know, like her brother and sister, grandmother and cousins, so she just kept the whole thing a secret.

What Dee didn't know was that her experience is a common one among high school and college-aged women. Most girls blame themselves for the rape or don't call it rape in the first place. They blame themselves for the same reasons Dee did: they were drinking or high, they allowed someone to come into their room or their apartment, they were being flirtatious or kissing them, or they did not protest or yell or say no enough. She didn't take into consideration that she reacted because she was afraid for her LIFE!

## Was This Date Rape?

Many young women will ask themselves, especially when this has happened at the hands of a person they know, even if they know him only casually, "Was this rape?" The following is a guide to answer that question.

### The Date Rape Test

- Did you give full consent or permission for sex?
- Were you drugged or too drunk to say yes?
- Did it involve betrayal of a trusted relationship?
- Was there violence or control over you?
- Did you feel abused?

According to sex therapist Wendy Maltz, if you say yes to any of these questions, chances are you were raped. You need to talk to a professional about these things. Most young women are scared to call something rape that they do not understand completely. Most young women feel it is their fault if a rape happens under these circumstances, and this IS WRONG. Many, many, many times as a therapist I have had to tell someone that, "Yes, that was rape." Even if you went to his apartment or even into his bedroom, that is not consent for sexual intercourse. Even if you became naked with him and were big time messing around, that is not consent for sexual intercourse. Or just because you are his girlfriend or fiancé or even his wife, that does not mean you have automatically consented to sex. Even husbands can be charged for raping their wives, because it is even illegal to force sex on your wife. Even marriage is not an agreement for sex that does not include one's permission at that moment. This offense is called Marital Rape.

## Drug Facilitated Sexual Assault

Date rape drugs can be used by sexual predators to drug women and rape them.

Three drugs are most commonly used for date or acquaintance rape:

1. GHB (gamma hydroxybutyric acid)
2. Rohypnol, also called "roofies"
3. Ketamine

Technically speaking, any drug or substance that makes you incapable of functioning or consenting to sexual contact can be used to commit rape. Alcohol, marijuana, ecstasy, over-the-counter sleeping pills and antihistamines, even cold medications can be used to make a girl incapacitated and unable to function. Anytime a person is unable to assert themselves and is too intoxicated or drugged to consent to sexual behavior, legally, it is considered rape. However, there are sexual predators who use drugs to make a victim unconscious and to sexually assault them. These date rape drugs are fast acting, tasteless, odorless, and colorless. They leave the body in 72 hours and are undetectable, unless the victim is tested very quickly and specifically for date rape drugs, leaving the victim with no memory of what happened to them.

In most situations, an unsuspecting victim suddenly feels very drunk or intoxicated, even when they have had little or nothing to drink. The drugs makes a victim, initially, act drunk and drugged, having little inhibitions, and later, unconscious or passed out. A victim may wake up with little or no memory of what happened to them. Often, the best evidence of being drugged comes from gossip from other people who report the victim was "very drunk," or acting "totally wasted." Other evidence of rape may come from signs of a sexual assault, such as defensive bruising or scratching, bodily fluids in one's body or on clothing, a used condom, or genital soreness.

## Protecting Yourself from Date Rape Drugs

- Don't accept drinks from other people
- If you're in a bar, only take drinks directly from the bartender and/or watch your drink coming directly to you. Don't let someone get a drink for you.
- Keep your drink with you all the time, never leave your drink unattended, even if you go to the bathroom
- Don't share drinks
- Open containers yourself
- Don't drink from punch bowls or from "trash can" party drinks
- Don't drink anything that tastes or smells strange or is salty (a sign of GHB)
- Have a "drinking buddy" or non-drinking friend with you to make sure nothing happens to either one of you
- If you or a friend seems to get very drunk, very fast, leave the party or bar immediately and together.

- For extra protection, you can buy drug test kits to test your drinks for date rape drugs at drinksafetech.com

- If you have gotten drunk very fast or you think you have been drugged:
    1. Go to the hospital right away
    2. Wait to go to the bathroom and get a urine (pee) test immediately
    3. Don't bathe or change clothes: they can be evidence
    4. Call a crisis line to talk to someone, such as National Domestic Hotline at 800–799-SAFE or the Teen NineLine at 1-800-999-9999.
    5. Get counseling help. Many girls feel guilty or ashamed, but it is not your fault and you should not be alone. Get help quickly!

## Acquaintance Rape with Emotional Coercion or Blackmail

If there is coercion for sex, this is rape. There is most obviously coercion when there is a physical threat, such as having a knife or gun held on you. There is also, and much more commonly, emotional coercion. In the following example, the young woman did know her rapist, so this was "acquaintance rape" that involved emotional coercion for sex.

## Elise's Story

Elise was a senior in high school. Elise considered herself to be a "liberated" young woman—progressive in her outlook on morality and politics. She liked sex and had enjoyed safe and responsible sex with a few previous sexual partners during the past 2 years. All of the relationships were mutual and consensual. She had used condoms and birth control faithfully and felt quite good about her sexuality. Elise enjoyed pleasure with these sexual encounters, which did not all include sexual intercourse, and she had had a variety of dating relationships with young men in her life. She had felt better about the longer-term relationships, but she considered the other relationships "learning experiences," including one "one night stand."

Elise began befriending a young man from her neighborhood named "Billy." Due to their backgrounds and their parents' friendship, they became friends very quickly. Billy knew Elise's parents. He knew that they had a very conservative view of sex and that they thought Elise was a virgin. Elise felt comfortable with Billy and talked to him about sex, and they both discussed their sexual histories.

Billy and Elise hung out together and talked a lot over one summer. One night, they went driving around and Billy was smoking weed. Billy liked Elise and he wanted to have sex with her. He thought she might be "easy" because of her sexual history, and he thought that he had a chance for some casual sex, even though he didn't have a romantic relationship with her. He asked Elise to have sex with him and Elise said no. She was not attracted to Billy and she just wanted to be friends. They had never had any kind of romantic or physical relationship, and Elise didn't want one with him.

After Elise turned Billy down for sex during this car ride, Billy became increasingly angry toward Elise. Then he became sexually aggressive toward her. He parked the car, which was a considerable distance from their neighborhood. Billy continued to try to convince Elise to have sex with him, and he began to physically make the moves on Elise, while she continued to say no to Billy. She forced his hands off her and demanded that he drive her home.

Then the emotional coercion came into play. Billy threatened to tell Elise's parents that she wasn't a virgin and to tell them about every guy she had sex with since she was 16 unless she had sex with him. Elise pleaded with him to just take her home and to not say anything to her parents. As with many teenagers, Elise's relationship with her parents had already been rocked by minor rebellions and conflicts and Elise did not want any further trouble with her parents. Also, she did not want her parents to judge her badly and then "never let her out of the house again," which she was certain would be their response if Billy betrayed her trust and told them everything.

Billy persisted, mocking Elise with the information that she had previously trusted him with about her personal life. Billy became very verbally aggressive with his threats and flatly refused to drive Elise home unless she had sex with him. Finally, feeling emotionally threatened, Elise agreed to have sex with Billy in the back seat of his car. Billy was forceful and rough, hurting her arms while he forced himself on her. The sexual intercourse hurt, too. Then he drove her home. He never did tell her parents anything.

Elise was raped by a young man wielding emotional coercion as a weapon. She did not know whether or not it was rape because she actually did agree to have sexual intercourse with him. However, this rape led to Elise having a deep depression. She later attempted suicide because she didn't trust the world or herself. What Elise experienced was coercive rape and acquaintance rape.

ALL rape is traumatic, but there is something particularly traumatic about a woman being raped by someone she knows and had previously liked and trusted. It can make you stop trusting all men and the whole world . . . at least for a while. For some people, that lack of trust and dislike of men can last for many years.

# On Rape: It Is Rape If You Don't Say No, Even If:

- You are emotionally forced by threat to say yes.

- He is horny and "needs some" and you are both naked and have done everything else but intercourse, but you didn't say yes.

- You have had sex before 100 times, but you didn't say yes this time

- You've had oral sex, but you didn't say yes to intercourse.

- It is your only opportunity for sex because . . . but you didn't say it was OK.

- You are married, but you didn't say yes.

- You are "dressed for sex."

- You have already had an orgasm and he hasn't.

- You invited him into your apartment, dorm room, or bedroom.

- You have been flirtatious.

- You have been his girlfriend for a whole year.

- You promised him, but you changed your mind.

Young women from 15–25 are particularly vulnerable to this type of sexual assault. Not all of these behaviors are preventable . . . but the rest of this chapter is devoted to providing information so that your risk might be reduced. Although date rape and acquaintance rape are not completely preventable, there are many things you can learn to do that may help to prevent you from becoming a victim. The following information is adapted from a booklet written by Jean Hughes and Bernice Sandler for the Project on the Status and Education of Women. The booklet was written for college-aged women to help them prevent date rape.

### How Does Date Rape Happen?

Date rape happens when a woman is alone with a man. If you go to a man's room or apartment or bring him to your room or apartment, you are vulnerable. Sometimes, date rapes happen when people are close by, such as when you are in an upstairs bedroom in a house when there is a loud party on the first floor.

Alcohol and drugs are often a big factor in date rape. Often, victims say later that they drank too much, like Dee, or took too many drugs to realize what was going on; by the time they realized the situation they were in, it was too late. Sometimes, like in Dee's situation, a woman awakens to find a man having sexual intercourse with her. At times, this can happen after she passes out. Date rapes do happen without drugs or alcohol, too, however.

Mixed up communication can happen in date rape. Sometimes, a woman acts friendly, and the man takes this as an invitation for sex. Sometimes a woman says "no" and a man hears "maybe." For some men, even a strong "no" can be ignored, as some men think women say no when they mean yes. If a woman protests mildly, some men find it sexually exciting for a women to struggle, and he may think he is merely "persuading" her to have sex, not forcing her to have sex. He may even think the same way when she is protesting strongly. Sometimes a woman is not clear in her own mind about what she wants, or she may think she will make up her mind as she goes along. If she changes her mind at some point and decides not to have sex, the man can feel cheated, rejected, or angry. He may be interpreting her nonverbal messages, such as her enjoyment of kissing and caressing, as meaning that she wants to have sex with him. At this point, a man may decide he has been teased or misled and "deserves" to get some sexual satisfaction, regardless of the woman's wishes. The result can be rape.

Although acquaintance rape is often a spontaneous act, many are planned, some days in advance, and others in the proceeding hour(s). Sometimes men plan to have sex with a woman even if they have to force the issue. These men often have forced sex on a woman before and gotten away with it. They usually look for victims who are unassertive—perhaps someone who is not very popular and would be flattered to go on a date with him. Needless to say, these men do not see themselves as repeat rapists; in their own minds, they are merely "out to have a good time."

## What Causes Date Rape?

There is no one cause of date rape. One major reason for it occurring is a man's lack of consideration for the woman's rights and wishes. Part of this is a problem with our society and how boys are taught to be men. Males are taught from a young age to be aggressors. They are taught in movies, in video games, and in sports to have sexual feelings and to express these feelings as part of being a man. Our society promotes a belief to men that they "have a right to have sex." Women, on the other hand, are taught more than not to avoid conflict, to go along with the flow, to be "ladylike" and not experiment or express their sexuality. Women are often categorized as either "virgins" or "whores" or as "good" or "promiscuous" with no middle ground. Men are encouraged to get laid—as soon as possible.

Communication between men and women is often a problem, especially when it comes to sex. This is perhaps especially true in the first sexual situation between a new couple: some women say "no" to be "good" so they won't be "whores" when they DO mean "maybe" or "I want to, but . . . " Men have been taught to try to change that "no/maybe/I want to, but . . . " into a yes. Most young men nowadays have learned a valuable lesson and know that if a woman says "no" and they continue anyway that is rape. But many of these same men think that it is OK to keep their hands and mouth moving to get a woman to say yes. Also, many women want to mess around with kissing and touching, including touching of their breasts, buttocks, and genitals, or having oral sex, but they don't want to have sexual intercourse.

These types of signals of a girl's willingness to be sexual in non-intercourse ways can lead some men to think that sexual intercourse is OK too. Such a situation is also one that fosters sexual assaults.

Some men believe (and women do, too!) that if a guy spends a lot of money on date, they are entitled to have sex. Some men (and women) believe that if they have gone out a few times, sex is expected. Some men believe that if they have had sex with a women once, they will get it again and again, since they have "crossed that line already." Some men believe that if a woman has been sexually active, she is willing to have sex with anyone she dates, including him.

Acquaintance rape is not only a crime of momentary passion or miscommunication. It is also an attempt to assert power and anger as well as sexual desire. Sometimes men assert sexual power because they are sexually frustrated or sexually insecure. Forcing sex on someone satisfies their sexual needs, but it also satisfies their needs to feel strong and to make someone else feel weak.

> Rape is violence against a woman: People who respect each other do not force others to do things they do not want to do.

## What You Can Do To Avoid Situations That Might Lead To Date Rape

First, you can't always avoid rape. Thinking that you can will only make you blame yourself if rape happens to you. However, you can do some things to lower your risk of being raped:

**1. Develop a strong sexual voice!** Many women are taught to be shy and avoid conflict and not talk about their real feelings with partners. This is especially true when it comes to talking about sex. This is your BODY! Use your own strength and your own voice to speak up and state clearly and firmly what you want and what you don't want. Don't even get close to having sex with anyone with whom you cannot express yourself, and the same holds true regarding anyone who does not respect you in non-sexual ways. If you can't communicate with respect outside the bedroom, chances are that you will have a lot of trouble doing it inside the sexual arena. Learn to communicate your feelings, become friends, be comfortable with who you are, and feel respected for your choice so that when it comes to sex you can speak up. Talk about your sexual feelings . . . LONG before you get into an intimate or isolated situation with your potential partner. Make sure he or she listens to you!

2. **Set sexual limits.** It is your body. No one has the right to force you to do anything you do not want to do. If you do not want someone to touch you or kiss you, for example, you can say, "Take your hands off me," or "Don't touch me," or "If you don't listen to me right now, I'm leaving." Stopping sexual activity does not mean there is anything wrong with you or that you are not a sexy, hot "real" woman. It merely means that this situation is not right for you in regard to sex.

3. **Decide early if you would like to have sex.** The sooner you tell your partner firmly and clearly your sexual intentions, the easier it will be for him to accept your decision.

4. **Don't give mixed messages.** Say "yes" when you mean "yes" and "no" when you mean "no."

5. **Be alert to other unconscious messages you may be giving.** Men may see your behavior differently than you intended. Watch out for signals that you send off via your

posture, body language, clothing, tone of voice, touch, and gestures. You do not want to mistakenly convey a willingness that is not genuine or real.

6. **Be forceful and firm.** Don't worry about being nice or "polite." Often men interpret quietness as permission. Say something like, "Stop this. I'm not enjoying it," or "What you are doing is turning me off, and I don't like it!" If a woman ignores a sexual activity that she does not like, men may interpret it as an approval for him to keep going. Men are not mind readers.

7. **Don't do anything you don't want to do to just avoid a scene or unpleasantness or so he will like you.** Do not be raped because you were too polite to get out of a dangerous situation. If you are worried about hurting his feelings, remember: HE IS IGNORING YOUR FEELINGS. It is OK to get angry; don't let yourself be vulnerable and go along with something so he will like you.

8. **If things start to get out of hand, despite your protests, leave and look for help.** If things start feeling uncomfortable and your requests for change are not working: Get out quickly.

9. **Trust your gut feelings.** If you feel you are being pressured, you probably are, and you need to respond to these feelings as soon as possible. If a situation feels bad or you start to get nervous about the way your date is acting, immediately confront the person or leave as soon as possible. Listen to your gut. It is your emotional alarm system. It turns on for a reason. It is better to feel "stupid" later for running away than to risk being raped. If you just don't feel things are right and your date is not making you feel any better

after talking about it, then leave. You can discuss it more rationally later, and you can apologize if you decide ultimately that your intuition was wrong.

10. **Carefully consider the possible consequences of drug and alcohol use while dating.** Don't allow your drinking or drugging to impair your judgment or turn off your natural alarm system (your gut feelings).

11. **Have your own transportation on early dates.** Meet for a first date during the day, like for lunch. Then meet him somewhere for the next one or two dates. After that, go to places where you can catch a cab or call a friend if you feel uncomfortable.

12. **Be careful about inviting someone to your home or going to someone else's home.** These are the most common places where acquaintance rapes take place. I cannot tell you how important it is to watch out for bedrooms at parties, too.

13. **Examine your attitudes toward money and power.** If he pays for the date, does that influence your ability to say "no?" If so, then pay you own way or suggest dates that do not involve money.

14. **Think about the pros and cons about dating much older men.** Although they may be more mature and sophisticated and have the money to treat you well, they may also be more sexually experienced and may therefore expect more from you sooner in terms of sexual behavior.

15. **Socialize with people who share your values.** If you go out with people who are more sexually permissive than you, it is likely that they will think you have the same values.

## An Alternative Male Perspective of Date Rape—Tim's Story

**When Tim was 14, he was hanging out with this girl, "Martha." Although nothing happened between Tim and Martha, Martha told two of her cousins that Tim molested her. The next thing Tim knew, these cousins happened to see him leaving a store. The two cousins accused Tim of "molesting" Martha, although they didn't say specifically what he had supposedly done to Martha. The two large, older, guys grabbed Tim and beat him to a bloody pulp. He was cut under his eye, bleeding all over his face, had a broken and bloody nose, two black eyes, and had to stagger home. Then Tim had to see his mother. He told her some guys jumped him for no reason and that he never ever came close to kissing or touching Martha. Tim didn't even like Martha. This really messed with Tim's feelings toward girls. He acted a lot more cautious about being alone with a girl, even though he had done nothing wrong.**

To be fair to guys, it is important to include in this chapter the fact that sometimes girls do lie about rape or sexual assault, including sexual molestation. Because rape is such an emotionally charged issue, and a crime, the accusation of rape can really get a young man into trouble. One of the problems with false accusations is that often a guy is guilty until proven innocent. Generally, no one believes the guy. This can happen in child sexual assault cases, although it has only been proven to happen less than 10% of the time. While that is a relatively small number, for the innocent person who is accused and assumed guilty, such a situation will have devastating effects on their lives.

### Why Girls Lie about Sexual Assault

- To get attention.
- To get out of admitting they agreed to have sex. I knew a 16 year-old girl who accused her boyfriend of rape because she did not want to admit to her father that she got caught with her boyfriend

in her bedroom, when in fact she invited him to be there.

- To not feel guilty about consenting to sex.
- To get some guy in trouble or generally hurt them.
- For revenge, like if the guy rejects her or doesn't call when he has said he will.
- When a girl changes her mind later about having sex, like the next day, then calls it rape.
- To achieve power.
- Some mothers have falsely accused their ex-husbands of child sexual assault to get child custody or to take away his visitation rights.

## Danger Signals of Rapists

Unfortunately, there are no specific "LOOKS" that a rapist has. A nice, normal looking guy can turn into a date rapist. However, there are some men who are more likely to be sexually aggressive than others. Watch out for:

1. Men who do not listen to you, ignore what you say, talk over you, or pretend not to hear you. These guys generally do not have much respect for women and would be more likely to hear "no" as meaning "convince me."
2. Men who ignore your personal space boundaries: they sit too close or put their arm around you too tightly, or grab your breast "just for a joke."
3. Men who express anger or aggression toward women as individuals or in general. Hostile feelings can lead to hostile acts. Such men often get hostile when a woman says "no."
4. Men who do what they want to do regardless of what you want. If a man does this in little ways—for example, he makes all the decisions about what to do and where to go without asking your opinion—then he may also be likely to make the decision about whether or not you are ready to have sex with him, too.

5. Men who try to make you feel guilty about your sexual values or morals, or accuse you of being "uptight" or "frigid" if you resist sexual advances.

6. Men who act excessively jealous or possessive. These kinds of men, at first, seem extremely loving, loyal, attentive and caring. But after a while, they are controlling . . . PERIOD. These type of men want to tell you what to wear, how to spend your money, who to have as friends, to limit your relationships with family, or they accuse you of looking at someone the "wrong way." They may be controlling about your home, dress, money, friends, work, or activities. Men who are controlling in these ways will be controlling about sex, too.

7. Men who have strong stereotypically sexist or unrealistic ideas about women. For example, "women are meant to have sex for men." These types of men are not likely to take your objections to sex seriously.

8. Men who drink or use drugs heavily. A "mean drunk" can often get sexually aggressive, angry, or violent if he is rejected. Some drugs, like Ecstasy, increase the sex drive. This extra boost to the sex drive can contribute to sexually aggressive behavior.

9. Men with a history of sexual assault.

### What Should You Do If Someone Tries to Force Sexual Activity?

1. Stay calm and think. Unfortunately, this is like keeping dry in a hurricane. Try to consider your options and how safe it is to resist.

2. Say "no" strongly. Do not smile, and do not act friendly or polite.

3. Say something like "Stop it. This is RAPE." This might shock your potential rapist into stopping.

4. Look at the situation. Figure out how you might escape. Are there any other people around?

5. Look for an escape route. If you can figure out a way to distract

him, you can sometimes escape. Do not let on that you want to get out of there. Do not alarm him. Act calm, like everything is OK, so that he is off guard.

6. Act quickly, if possible. The longer you stay in the situation, the fewer your options.

7. If he is drinking or drugging and the substances are not making him mean or sexually aggressive, suggest he have some more. If he gets higher or drunker, and you don't, you will have more control in the situation because you will be more alert and clear headed than he is. Suggest that you go get him a drink or a joint, which could also be an escape plan. His vice or addiction may temporarily distract him.

8. Ask yourself if it is safe to resist. This is a critical question. Women who fight back initially, who hit and scream, have a much higher chance of avoiding the successful completion of an assault than do women who plead or try to talk their way out of the situation. Nevertheless, resistance will depend on one main question: is he armed?

*If The Man Is Unarmed, Then You Have Many Options . . .*

- Fight back physically, punch him in the Adam's apple, poke your finger in his eye, kick him in the balls, hit him with a lamp or other items. Fight so that you can escape, as it is difficult for most women to incapacitate a man. Resistance may discourage the man or convince him that it's too much trouble to continue. Resist only as long as it is safe to do so. If resistance is dangerous, stop.
- Run away. There is no shame in escaping a dangerous situation.
- Say you have to use the bathroom.
- Shout "fire." If you shout "help," some people will tend not to want to be involved in someone else's problem. "Fire" concerns them and they are more likely to respond.
- Throw up.

What Every Girl Needs to Know About Rape and Sexual Abuse

- Gross him out: Urinate.
- Use intimidation, and lie if you have to: tell him your male room-mate is on the way home.
- Tell him you have a STD, like AIDS or herpes.
- Try to talk him out of it by appealing to his sense of decency.
- Be nice (after being firm and it doesn't work) and gain his confidence so that he lets down his and you can escape.
- Try to get him to see you as an individual person. Make him aware of the effect he is having on you. Tell him that he is hurting you.
- Tell him that you're having your period; some men are turned off by menstruation.

### If The Man Is Armed, Then . . .

- Try to talk him out of it; try especially to get him to see you as a person who is hurting because of what he is doing.
- Try passive resistance, such as urinating or throwing up.
- You are taking your life in your hands if you fight back, so be very careful about this.
- Try to run away, only if you are reasonably sure that you can get away.

### What to Do If You Are Raped

1. Go to a friend or family member. Do not be alone.
2. If one person does not believe you or want to be with you, try another, then another, if necessary.
3. Get medical attention. Tell them you were raped and make sure they use a rape kit.
4. Report the incident to the police.
5. Get professional counseling help.
6. DO NOT BLAME YOURSELF . . . NO MATTER WHAT!!!!

# Your Sexual Rights

This is your life, your sexuality, your body, and your future. Enjoy . . . but, take care of yourself and develop your sexual voice with as much determination and energy as you will need to protect your mind, body, and spirit. Remember that you have sexual rights and it is up to you to exercise them.

~~~~~~~~~~~~~~~~~~~~~~~~~~~~~~~~~~~~~~~~~~~~

The right to develop healthy attitudes about sex

~~~~~~~~~~~~~~~~~~~~~~~~~~~~~~~~~~~~~~~~~~~~

The right to sexual privacy

The right to protect yourself from bodily invasion and harm

The right to say no to sexual behavior

The right to control touch and sexual contact

The right to stop sexual excitement that feels inappropriate

The right to develop your sexuality according to your sexual preferences and orientation

The right to enjoy healthy sexual pleasure and satisfaction

(Reprinted with the permission of Wendy Maltz, MSW, AASECT Certified Sex Therapist)

273

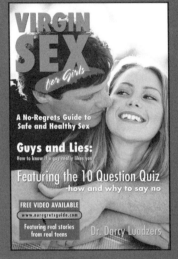

# About the Website

If *Virgin Sex for Girls* got you wondering what other teens thought of these topics, come visit our companion website, www.noregretsguide.com. There, you can download and view video clips of your peers discussing everything in this book—and more!

Short video clips can be downloaded right to your computer. Find out what other teens thought about the "Are You Ready for Sex?" Quiz, religious values and sex, birth control, date rape, having (and not having) sex, coming out, relationship lies, and the other topics covered in *Virgin Sex for Girls*.

While you're there, take the time to ask Dr. Darcy your own sex question, read and comment on Dr. Darcy's blog, and browse the archive of frequently asked questions and other resources. You can stay completely anonymous. If this book has left something unanswered, please come and ask. Join the conversation, learn more about safe and healthy sex, download videos of teens in open debate, and much more—it's all part of the community of teens at www.noregretsguide.com.

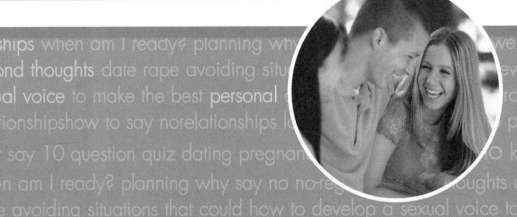

# Bibliography

Alanguttmacher.org. The Guttmacher Institute, New York and Washington, 2006.

Basso, Michael J. *The Underground Guide to Teenage Sexuality*. Fairview Press, 1997.

Bell, Ruth. *Changing Bodies, Changing Lives: A Book for Teens on Sex and Relationships*. Random House, 1998.

Dodson, Betty. *Sex for One: The Joy of Self Loving*. Random House, 1987.

Hughes, Jean, and Sandler, Bernice. *Friends Raping Friends*. Association of American Colleges, 1987.

Maltz, Wendy. *The Sexual Healing Journey*. HarperCollins Publishers, 1991.

Masters, W., Johnson, V. Human Sexual Response. Little, Brown, 1966.

Mosher, WD, Chandra, A, Jones, J. Sexual Behavior and selected health measures: Men and Women 15–44 years of age. United States, 2002. Advance data from vital and health statistics, no 367. Hyattsville, MD. National Center for Health Statistics, 2005.

Nakashima, AK, Rolfs, RT, Flock, ML, Kilmarx, P, Greenspan, JR. *Epidemiology of syphilis in the US 1941 through 1993*. Sexually Transmitted Diseases, 1196, 23:16--23.

National Child Exploitation Coordination Centre (NCECC). Internet Based Sexual Exploitation of Children and Youth Environmental Scan,

http://ncecc.ca/enviroscan_2005_e.htm, 2005.

National Center for Missing and Exploited Children. "Don't Believe the Type," 2006.

Planned Parenthood. *The Emergency Contraception Handbook*. Planned Parenthood Federation of America, March, 1999.

# Resource Listings

## Free Telephone Hotline Numbers

Adolescent Crisis Intervention & Counseling Nineline
1-800-999-9999

AIDS National Hotline
1-800-342-2437

Al-Anon/Alateen Hotline
1-800-344-2666

Alcohol/Drug Abuse Hotline
1–800–662-HELP

Be Sober Hotline
1–800-BE-SOBER

Child Abuse Hotline
1–800–4-A-CHILD

Cocaine Hotline
1–800-Cocaine

Domestic Violence Hotline
1-800-548-2722

Emergency Contraception Information
1–800-NOT-2-LATE

Family Violence
1-800-313-1310

Gay & Lesbian National Hotline
1–888-THE-GLNH (843-4564)

Gay, Lesbian, Bisexual, and Trangender (GLBT) Youth Support Line
1-800-850-8078

Help Finding a Therapist
1–800-THERAPIST

Homeless/Runaway National Hotline
1-800-231-6946

Incest Hotline for guys: M.A.L.E.
1–800–949-MALE

National Adolescent Suicide Hotline
1-800-621-4000

National Association for Children of Alcoholics
1–800–55–4CHOAS (1-888-554-2627)

National Abortion Federation Hotline
1-800-772-9100

National Adoption Center
1-800-648-4400

National Child Abuse Hotline
1-800-422-4453

National Drug Abuse Hotline
1–800–622-HELP

National STD Hotline
1-800-227-8922

National Youth Crisis Hotline
1-800-448-4663

National Victim Center
1–800-FYI-CALL

People Against Rape
   1-800-877-7252

Planned Parenthood
   1–800–230-PLAN

Pregnancy Hotline
   1–800–4-OPTIONS

Pregnant & Young Hotline (Birthright)
   1-800-550-4900

Rape, Abuse, Incest, National Network (RAINN)
   1–800–656-HOPE

Runaway Hotline
   1-800-231-6946

Safe Choice Hotline (STDs & Pregnancy)
   1-800-878-2347

Self-Injury Hotline
   1–800-DON'T-CUT

Sexual Assault Hotline
   1-800-656-4673

Stop it Now! (Sexual Abuse)
   1–800-PREVENT

TalkZone (Peer Counselors—other teens)
   1–800–475-TALK

TeenLine
   1-800-522-8336

The Trevor HelpLine (specializing in gay and lesbian youth suicide
prevention)
   1-800-850-8078

Youth Crisis Hotline
   1-800-448-4663
   1-800-422-0009

## Website Listings

**www.teenwire.com**
   Planned parenthood site for sexual health information

**www.drinksafetech.com**
   Info on drug testing kits for drinks to avoid drug facilitated sexually assault

**http://womensissues.about.com/od/rapecrisis/a/rapestats.htm**

# Index

283

284

Index